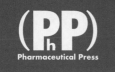

Conducting Your Pharmacy Practice Research Project

Third Edition

Sara Garfield
Felicity Smith

Published by the Pharmaceutical Press
66-68 East Smithfield, London E1W 1AW, UK

© Pharmaceutical Press 2020

(**Ph P**) is a trade mark of Pharmaceutical Press
Pharmaceutical Press is the publishing division of the Royal Pharmaceutical Society

First edition published 2005
Second edition published 2010
Third edition published 2020

Printed in Great Britain by TJ International, Padstow, Cornwall

ISBN 978 0 85711 393 1

A catalogue record for this book is available from the British Library.

TABLE OF CONTENTS

About the authors.. ii
Preface...iii

PART 1 PREPARATION, PLANNING AND MANAGEMENT
Chapter 1. Introduction..5
Chapter 2. Types of pharmacy practice projects.............................. 11
Chapter 3. Setting up the project, protocol development and ethics 17
Chapter 4. Time management and working with others..................................29
Chapter 5. Patient and public involvement...37
Chapter 6. For supervisors...47

PART 2 SCIENTIFIC ENQUIRY AND RESEARCH/SERVICE EVALUATION METHODOLOGY
Chapter 7. A scientific approach to your research.............................59
Chapter 8. Reviewing the literature...73
Chapter 9. Study design...89
Chapter 10. Sources of information, datasets, sampling and recruitment 101
Chapter 11. Data collection - survey research and questionnaires................. 121
Chapter 12. Data collection - interviews and focus groups............................. 137
Chapter 13. Data collection - prospective methods 153
Chapter 14. Existing datasets and secondary analyses 161

PART 3 WRITING UP AND DISSEMINATION OF FINDING
Chapter 15. Data processing and analysis 169
Chapter 16. Writing the project report/research paper.....................................195
Chapter 17. Dissemination of the findings 207

Answers...217
Index 225

About the authors

Dr Sara Garfield is a registered pharmacist with over 20 years of experience of conducting, leading and supervising pharmacy practice research projects at both undergraduate and postgraduate level. Following completion of her PhD identifying factors affecting patients' decisions about taking antidepressant medication, she has held a number of post-doc positions where she has been successful in applying for research grants and has published widely. She has led a wide range of pharmacy projects in both primary and secondary care settings including research, quality improvement, service evaluation and audit. She currently works at Imperial NIHR Patient Safety Translational Research Centre, where her role includes leading in expanding patient and public involvement in research. She won the NIHR Clinical Research Award in excellence in patient and public involvement in 2019. She is also the lead tutor for international master's students conducting their pharmacy practice projects at University College London School of Pharmacy.

Professor Felicity Smith is a registered pharmacist with experience of hospital and community pharmacy. After completing her PhD, evaluating the contribution of community pharmacists to primary healthcare in London at St Bartholomew's Hospital Medical College in London, she joined the academic staff of the School of Pharmacy, University College London where she is currently a Professor in its Department of Practice and Policy. Felicity Smith is experienced in the application of a wide range of health services research methodologies and tools in pharmacy settings.

Preface

The scope of pharmacy practice projects is huge. This is a reflection of the fact that, in order to promote safe and appropriate use of medicines, pharmacists have to take so many issues into account. New directions in health policy, changing needs and expectations of the population, the structural, economic, social and cultural contexts of healthcare, and the aspirations of pharmacists for a greater role in its delivery all provide the background and frameworks for the conception and execution of pharmacy practice research. Equally diverse is the range of approaches and methods that may be employed to answer important questions.

The projects conducted under the umbrella of 'pharmacy practice' is important to patients, carers, healthcare organisations, governments and the profession. The ultimate goal is to lead the way in the adaptation of pharmacy services to meet health and pharmaceutical care needs and contribute to pharmacy and health policy agendas.

Participation in original research is also seen as a fundamental component in a student's education. Professional bodies and national and international criteria for the award of professional and degree qualifications include descriptors relating to the understanding of principles of scientific enquiry and research methodology, the pursuit of scholarship, and the acquisition of research skills. Conducting or supervising a project should be seen as an opportunity not only to develop personal skills, but also to produce an original piece of work that has the potential to influence services of the future. However, it will be a challenging task as students will often be new to the settings and processes of their work.

This book is intended principally for less experienced researchers or supervisors. It provides an overview of the whole process of undertaking a project from initial planning and literature review through to the presentation of the final report and dissemination of findings.

This third edition of the text has been produced to reflect the major changes that have taken place in pharmacy practice projects and research in the last 10 years. The text has been comprehensively revised and expanded in recognition of the increased diversity of projects undertaken by students in the field of pharmacy practice, including service evaluation and audit, the rapidly growing role of technology in health services delivery and research, and the expansion of patients and public involvement in pharmacy practice projects. It includes many new sections, including the use of electronic data sets. The section on developing search terms in chapter 8 has been expanded with input from Peter Field, Information Skills Manager at UCL School of Pharmacy library.

Two new chapters have also been written. The first of these is designed to help students to recognise the type of project they are carrying out from the start of their project, allowing them to plan their methodology and applications for approvals. Secondly, the small section on patient and public involvement in the 2nd edition has been replaced by a full chapter giving a step by step guide to involving patients and the public in pharmacy practice projects in a meaningful and collaborative way. This chapter has been written in partnership with seven patient and public involvement representatives who have worked on pharmacy practice projects.

In addition to these changes, learning objectives and questions with answers have been added for all chapters to allow a more interactive approach including self-assessment of learning.

Sara Garfield
Felicity Smith
July 2020

CHAPTER 1

Introduction

LEARNING OBJECTIVES

Upon completion of this chapter you should be able to:

- describe the scope of pharmacy practice based research
- identify the value of conducting a pharmacy practice project to different stakeholders including patients, carers, healthcare professionals and policymakers.

What is pharmacy practice research?

The scope of pharmacy practice research is wide and rapidly expanding. It is used as an umbrella term for research into many different areas such medicines use, the pharmacy profession and pharmacy services. Topics relating to medicines use may include the medicines related beliefs and behaviour of patients and their carers, healthcare professionals' prescribing, dispensing and administration practices, and the impact of technologies and systems such as electronic prescribing. Projects relating to the pharmacy profession cover education, regulation or workforce issues. Evaluations of pharmacy services include the assessment of existing services and the development and evaluation of new services.

Pharmacy practice research is commonly viewed as a branch of health services research. This is because, firstly, pharmacy services and medicines are integral to health care and need to be studied in the context of wider health care provision and practices. Secondly, the approaches and methods employed in pharmacy practice research are similar to those applied to other areas of health services research. As will be discussed in other chapters, researchers draw on a wide range of disciplines and methodologies to enable the complexities of the subject to be examined in their wider contexts.

A further attraction of pharmacy practice research is its value. Research is rarely undertaken only out of curiosity, but with a particular application in view. The ultimate goal is to improve services and promote the safe and effective use of medicines. Pharmacy practice research is important to patients, carers, the pharmacy profession and other practitioners, health care organisations, policymakers and governments. Research should inform the development of pharmacy services, providing an evidence base for service development. It can identify ways in which services can most effectively meet the pharmaceutical care needs of their communities and contribute to health policy and priorities.

Researchers from pharmacy, medicine, epidemiology, sociology, anthropology, psychology, history and economics, among others, have applied themselves to studies of pharmacy services and the use of medicines. This has stimulated many within the discipline of pharmacy to incorporate different approaches and methods into addressing pharmacy related problems. Collaboration between pharmacists, other health professionals, special interest groups, voluntary organisations, consumers and/or members of the public is also a common feature of this research.

Throughout the world, reforms in the organisation and delivery of health care feature on governments' agendas. In addition, there are continually new approaches to, and medicines for, the management of disease. The ever evolving health policies and priorities present new opportunities and challenges for pharmacy. We must be prepared to review our practices critically, to innovate to meet the changing contexts of service provision, to respond to increased public expectations and health policy directions.

It's your project

Participation in original research is seen as a fundamental part of studies for a Masters' or higher degree. It is usually undertaken towards the final stages of an undergraduate pharmacy programme. The professional accreditation requirements for a pharmacy degree and nationally and internationally accepted criteria for the award of a Masters or higher degree include descriptors relating to the understanding of research methodology, the acquisition of research skills and their application to an individual research project (*Box 1.1*). These statements (which translate into learning objectives) will differ between universities, but they provide a broad indication of what you are expected to achieve. You may like to reflect on your achievement of these goals during the course of your project work.

> **Box 1.1: Typical learning objectives that should be achieved at Master's level**
>
> - A systematic understanding of knowledge and a critical awareness of current problems or new insights at the forefront of your discipline.
> - A conceptual understanding that enables you to critically evaluate current research, scholarship and methodologies.
> - A practical understanding of how established techniques of research are used to create and interpret new knowledge in your discipline.
> - A comprehensive understanding of techniques applicable to your own research.

For project work undertaken by students the responsibilities for different aspects of the research will be shared with their supervisors. How this is shared will depend on the nature and complexity of the project, its place in a wider research programme and your experience and ideas. There is a chapter which provides some suggestions on how this partnership might work, and the respective roles and responsibilities of students and supervisors (see **Chapter 6**). However, it is important that you make the project your own. Even if the objectives and methods have all been decided (which is often the case) you should make sure that you understand how and why these have been specified, that you are able to describe how the study fits into, and or adds to, the wider literature, comment on the strengths and weaknesses of methods and possibly any alternative approaches. If you are involved in the data collection and analysis, you may have to make some of your own decisions regarding how you will deal with any unexpected events or problems (which arise in most research projects) or check on the reliability and validity of the methods and findings. You should also be making decisions about how to analyse data and the interpretation of the findings, writing your project discussion and drawing conclusions.

Conducting a pharmacy practice project should be seen as a valuable experience that requires bringing together intellectual, organisational and administrative skills. Many projects provide an opportunity to participate in an original piece of work that has the potential to inform services in the future. Whether the goal of your project is to apply a theoretical approach that may further our conceptual understanding, or a structured evaluation of existing practices (e.g. audit), you need to adopt a scientific approach to all stages of the work.

The pharmacy practice project chapters aim to provide you with a guide to conducting your research project from the early planning stages through to submitting a high quality project report.

The preparation, planning and management chapters set the scene and focus on planning the work, organisational aspects of the project, its management and execution. You will have a finite length of time for your project work. If you want to achieve a high quality piece of work you must use your time effectively. Careful planning with realistic goals and clear milestones regarding what you should aim to achieve at time points throughout will help ensure that you work as efficiently as possible. In any research project you must be prepared for busy and less busy times. When you are waiting for the project work to commence or if you have a period during which you cannot proceed with fieldwork, you should make sure that you use the time productively.

Many projects will be collaborative. In your project work you may well require the cooperation and involvement of others, especially if you are working in a professional environment. Research is commonly a shared endeavour. Whilst you have to take ultimate responsibility for your work, there are parts of this book which provide some guidance on what to expect when working with others, including patients and members of the public (see **Chapter 4**). There is also a chapter for supervisors (see **Chapter 6**), who although are often experienced professionals, may be new to the supervision of student projects or unfamiliar with the requirements of degree programmes and universities.

The scientific enquiry and research methodology chapters are concerned with the principles of scientific enquiry and research methodology. This commences with a chapter on the nature and diversity of approaches to scientific enquiry applied to research into aspects of health services, medicines use and professional practice. Subsequent chapters focus on research design and types of study, data sources and principles of sampling, data collection and research instruments, data processing and analysis.

The writing up and dissemination of the findings chapters focus on writing up, presentation and dissemination of the study findings. Researchers hope that their work will inform future practice and contribute to improvements in service provision, patient care and health outcomes. Many projects that are undertaken as part of a Master's degree contribute to a wider research programme, or produce outcomes that have an application in informing practice at a local level. The project report should be written to a high standard and include all relevant information and methodological detail so it can be used a basis for wider discussion and dissemination.

Dissemination of findings is viewed as a crucial element in the research process. Work that does not reach interested stakeholders is unlikely to contribute to current debates or influence service development, and may be viewed as a waste of effort and resources. The final chapter discusses the preparation of summaries, reports or presentations for a variety of audiences.

Questions

1. **Which of the following would be pharmacy practice research projects? (Select all which apply)**
   A: Evaluating the opinions of patients on the pharmacy service
   B: Exploring the training needs of practitioners involved in pharmacy education
   C: Evaluating the effectiveness of the therapeutic drug monitoring of a high-risk medication in a hospital
   D: Evaluating the effects of the introduction of electronic prescribing system on medication errors
   E: Identifying the interventions made by general practice-based pharmacists
   F: Evaluating the proportion of patients on non-steroidal anti-inflammatories that are prescribed a gastroprotective medicine.

2. **Briefly list pharmacy practice research projects that you have read about or been involved with, highlighting the diversity in their scope.**

CHAPTER 2

Types of pharmacy practice projects

LEARNING OBJECTIVES

Upon completion of this chapter you should be able to:

- describe the different categories of pharmacy practice projects
- distinguish between research, service evaluation and audit.

Pharmacy practice projects differ in their goals and purpose, application of scientific enquiry, research design and methodology. Pharmacy projects generally fall under three categories: audit, service evaluation or research. There are many similarities between these in terms of the need for a scientific robust approach and the methods employed. It is not always easy to decide which category projects fall into due to many overlapping features between them. However, it is important to identify which type of project yours is so that you can frame it appropriately. This will also have implications for ethics approval (see **Chapter 3**).

Research

Research is the diligent and systematic inquiry or investigation into a subject in order to discover or revise facts, theories and applications. Research will involve an original investigation undertaken in order to enhance general knowledge and understanding of a subject with application beyond that of the local setting that it is carried out in.

Service evaluation

The aim of many studies is to evaluate either an aspect of current practice or a new service. Service evaluation is undertaken to benefit those who use a particular service and is designed and conducted to define or judge current service. The participants will normally be those who use the service or deliver it.

The scope and range of services offered by pharmacists are developing fast. Examples include the development of clinical services in general practice surgeries and growing roles in chronic condition management. Many pharmacists are committed to extending and improving the services that they offer. They also recognise the need to assess which developments meet the needs of the public or patients and will work in a practice setting.

An evaluation study will often focus on two areas. First, when a new service is introduced this will usually be with very specific objectives in mind (often related to improvements in some aspect of patient care). Thus, the evaluation will include an assessment of whether or not (and the extent to which) the new service has achieved its intended effect, possibly also comparing outcomes with usual care. Second, changes to service provision may also present problems, some of which may not be anticipated. When evaluating a service development, potential problems must also be identified. These may relate to its workability in different practice settings, its acceptability to health professionals, other staff or clients, logistical problems in its implementation and the costs of provision and/or cost-effectiveness, etc.

Thus, an evaluation may assess the following:

- The effectiveness of a service in terms of its principal and secondary outcomes.
- The feasibility: is the intervention workable for the professionals involved, and acceptable to clients and other stakeholders? What problems arise in its implementation?

As well as providing information about the extent of the effectiveness and feasibility of a service, the reasons why a service is succeeding or failing will also be evaluated. Investigating questions such as why it may be successful in some areas and not others, and how any barriers may be overcome can then be used to inform service improvement.

Audit

Audit is a much more specific measurement of the performance against predetermined specific standards. Audit uses research methods to monitor, evaluate and improve processes and outcomes. The design of an audit is according to the 'audit cycle'. An audit involves gathering information on an aspect of healthcare, service delivery, professional practice or the use of medicines and comparing this to predetermined standards or guidelines. In the first instance, the subject and aims of the audit are specified. These typically relate to some identified priority or problem regarding an aspect of service delivery or patient outcomes. Data are then collected to document current practices (c.f. a descriptive study). Following this, an assessment is made regarding the extent to which the standards are met, and any changes or interventions that are needed to either address deficiencies in practice or to improve standards. The audit process is then repeated. Standards may be redefined and then a further assessment performed. Thus, the design of audit is illustrated by the audit cycle or spiral (*Figure 2.1*).

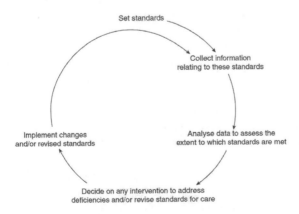

Figure 2.1: *The audit cycle or spiral*

The goal of audit is to generate information which can be used to document and improve an organisation's processes and outcomes. It is seen as an indispensible activity for organisations involved in the provision of healthcare.

The differences between research, service evaluation and audit

Table 2.1 summarises the difference between research, service evaluation and audit. Research, audit and service evaluation all use a range of health service research methodologies. However, the aims and objectives will determine which type of project it is. A research project will aim to tell us what best practice is, whereas an audit will tell us to what extent we are achieving accepted standards. A service evaluation will aim to produce internal recommendations for service development or improvement, whereas a research project will aim to generate generalisable findings and produce external recommendations. While a service evaluation may also inform external recommendations and a research project may also produce internal recommendations, they will differ as to which of these is their primary aim.

It is perhaps on a conceptual level that audit and service evaluation is distinguished from research. Audit does not generally draw on or aim to extend existing conceptual frameworks or theory. The knowledge generated will usually be of direct practical rather than theoretical application. Audit focuses on the documentation of current activity and achievements rather than questioning, developing and testing potential new approaches. A goal of audit is not to contribute to scholarship within a discipline or to provide new perspectives on an existing evidence base. However, audit requires a systematic approach to gathering data that is a valid and reliable reflection of the processes and outcomes of interest. To achieve this sampling strategies and procedures, data collection, data analysis and interpretation have to be undertaken to a standard of methodological rigour similar to research.

Whilst many projects can clearly be categorised as either research, audit or service evaluation, in some situations the distinction is less clear. An audit may provide use background information at the planning stages of a research study. In some audits, although conducted locally, the findings may be argued as having a wider relevance. Many research studies are confined to single sites. In some cases an audit or service evaluation may draw on an existing theoretical or explanatory framework which will inform its design and execution.

A key difference between an audit and a service evaluation is that an audit will measure performance against guidelines or an agreed predefined set of standards, whereas service evaluation will not measure against specific standards.

Another factor to consider is whether the project will involve any changes to patients' usual care such as treatment or additional procedures. If so, the project is likely to be classified as research from an ethics point of view (see **Chapter 3**).

Table 2.1: *Features of research, service evaluation and audit*

	Research	Service evaluation	Audit
Aims	To create new knowledge, concepts or theories	To evaluate an existing or new service	To evaluate to what extent practice is in line with recommendations
Procedures	May involve changes to existing treatments or invasive procedures	Will not involve changes to existing treatments of invasive procedures	Will not involve changes to existing treatments or invasive procedures
Ethics approvals required	NHS ethics approval required if it involves patients or NHS staff	Local approvals may be needed	Local approvals may be needed

Questions

1. **Which of the following is most likely to be a service evaluation?**
   A: Testing the extent to which a self-administration policy is being followed in a hospital trust
   B: Exploring patients' views on the self-administration in a hospital trust, with a view to improving the service at the hospital
   C: Identifying barriers to self-administration in the inpatient setting

2. **Which of the following is most likely to be an audit?**
   A: Determining whether there is an association between gentamycin dosing and nephrotoxicity
   B: Identifying the extent to which dosing guidelines for gentamcyin are followed in a hospital trust
   C: Determining the effects on the gentamycin dosing regime followed at a hospital trust on its patients' outcomes

3. **What distinguishes research from service evaluation?**

4. **Name the steps in the audit cycle.**

5. **Evaluation of a service may focus on effectiveness in terms of outcomes, or feasibility in terms of operation. With reference to your study or another service, explain these two aspects.**

CHAPTER 3

Setting up the project, protocol development and ethics

LEARNING OBJECTIVES

Upon completion of this chapter you should be able to:

- describe the processes needed to set up a pharmacy practice project
- develop aims and objectives for a pharmacy practice project
- identify and address ethical issues arising from a pharmacy project.

Planning a project thoroughly is key to its success. While all projects are different, most will have several stages including:

- a literature review and/or background reading
- some preliminary fieldwork to identify a gap in knowledge that the project will fill
- the development of aims and smart objectives for the project
- the development of methods and methodology that will allow the researcher to meet the aims and objectives
- data collection
- data analysis
- dissemination and impact related activities.

Investing time and effort in the preparatory stages of a project is usually immensely worthwhile and the identification of relevant and achievable objectives ensure feasible, acceptable and effective methodology to succeed in meeting these aims. The development of a project protocol which provides an overview of the rationale for, and the operation of, the project can be very helpful in planning. For many projects, some form of approval must be obtained before the work can commence and the project must meet requirements regarding data protection regulations, confidentiality and other legal and ethical issues. A project protocol which includes a description of the methods enables the identification of actual, or potential, ethical issues, which can then be addressed.

Preparing a protocol

Many projects commence with the development of a 'protocol'. This provides a detailed plan of all the stages of the project: its conception, aims and research question, the methods and procedures that will be employed, anticipated outcomes and information regarding the timeline, costs/resources and management (*Box 3.1*). The protocol should provide sufficient detail to allow a researcher to carry out the project and will be referred to and followed throughout its duration.

The protocol will often be informed by a literature review and preliminary fieldwork. These help in identifying key issues and refining research questions, and selecting the most appropriate methods. Together they lead to the development of the protocol.

Box 3.1: A research protocol

This may include the following:

- Introduction: provides the background to the project, the rationale for undertaking the research, followed by a statement of aims and objectives (or research question). The introduction should show how the project will build on existing knowledge, provide new information to fill an important gap in knowledge and/or contribute to service development.
- Methods: an explanation of the methodological approach and design of the study. The methods and procedures that will be employed should be detailed. This should include some justification for their selection and comments on how potential problems will be addressed. Separate sections may include details of sampling procedures, recruitment of participants, methods of data collection, research instruments and other documentation (e.g. questionnaires, data collection forms, information leaflets, consent forms) and plans for the analysis of data.
- Details of the programme of work including: timescales, project milestones, management processes and anticipated outcomes.

Literature review

A review of the literature is a requirement in many degree programmes. It is commonly undertaken prior to, or in the early stages of project work. This is often expected to be a comprehensive piece of work, applying a systematic approach. Thus, a chapter is devoted to reviewing the literature (see **Chapter 8**). New projects should build on previous work and take into account factors that are already known or thought to be important to the subject of study. A review of the literature identifies earlier studies in the subject area, thus providing researchers with an insight into what is already known about a topic and relevant factors to take into account in their own work. The review may also uncover pertinent issues that have not been formally investigated by researchers, but have been reported anecdotally as important. In terms of methodology, previous researchers will describe the methods that they used to collect data or measure important variables. This information may be helpful to you when deciding your methods and procedures. It is, of course, important to acknowledge your sources fully to avoid risks of plagiarism.

What is preliminary fieldwork?

Preliminary fieldwork enables the researcher to ensure that the important issues from the perspective of the population of interest, or characteristics of the setting are identified. Thus, if the goal of the project is to assess the value of a new service from the perspective of health professionals and/ or clients, the researcher may at the start have some informal discussions with a few key individuals to gain some insights into their expectations and experiences. This would ensure that issues important to these stakeholders could be incorporated when developing the protocol. If a project were to be an audit of the use of particular medicines some preliminary fieldwork, to check on the extent of use of the medicines and/or how information could be obtained may be valuable for planning the project. For a study focusing on experiences of a patient group, before detailed methods can be written, you may need to know the number of patients that are eligible for the study, their location and/or possible ways of accessing the relevant data.

Many larger studies require a structured and scientific approach to preliminary fieldwork to enable an informed case for the larger project to be made (*Box 3.2*). The preliminary fieldwork is an important stage of the work. All aspects of the rationale for the study and the methods have to be supported in terms of the perceived need for the work and its relevance, the feasibility of the methods proposed and the likelihood of the anticipated outcomes being achieved. A student project may sometimes comprise the preliminary fieldwork for a larger study.

Box 3.2: The purpose and scope of preliminary fieldwork

- Assesses the importance of the research to various potential stakeholders and ensures that all their thoughts and concerns are identified and taken into account in designing the work
- Assists in the refinement of the aims and objectives
- Allows an exploration of the feasibility of different methodological approaches from the perspective of potential participants
- Informs the development of the research instruments
- Aids the preparation and review of documentation (information leaflets, data collection forms, etc.)

Preliminary fieldwork may involve informal discussions with interested parties, potential participants or their representatives. The aims will be, first, to ensure that the study objectives address the perspectives of these different groups and, second, that the methods and procedures of the study will be acceptable and workable. Preliminary fieldwork is sometimes designed to provide specific information required for the development of the protocol, e.g. for a study involving hospital staff or patients you may need to find information on the number of staff or size of hospital. Preliminary fieldwork can be invaluable for the ultimate success of a study. Discussing your proposal with interested individuals, who may have direct experience of the issues and problems and practicalities of conducting projects in a particular setting, can be immensely helpful, improving your awareness of the subject area and the potential problems.

Thus, the preliminary fieldwork, along with the literature review, help refine the study objectives and inform the choice of methods.

Specifying your aims and objectives

The aim of a study relates to its overall goal, whereas the objectives are specific and measurable; they detail how the aim is to be met. Objectives should be SMART wherever possible:

- Specific, i.e. well defined and clear
- Measurable, i.e. allow you to measure if, when and to what the extent the objectives are achieved
- Achievable, for example with the time and resources you have available
- Relevant to your project aim (the components of your objectives should lead to your project aim)
- Timely, i.e. time frame for achievement should be specified

The importance of having clear statements of the aims and objectives cannot be underestimated. They underpin decisions regarding the design of the study (e.g. whether it is experimental or descriptive), the type of sample that is needed, the data that will be required and the analytical procedures necessary to answer research questions and achieve specific objectives. Precision in the objectives is, therefore, vital to all stages of the work. A lack of clarity can result in an unfocused study that does not answer any research questions effectively. For example, for a project addressing lack of facilitation of self-administration of medicines in hospital for patients wanting it, the project aim might be:

- To develop and evaluate an intervention to make self-administration more easily available to hospital inpatients who wanted it.
- SMART objectives may then be:
  - To increase the proportion of all inpatients reporting being aware of the self-administration option within six months.
  - To increase the proportion of all inpatients recorded as self-administering medication within six months.
  - To increase the proportion of inpatients who wished to self-administer their medication who reported that they had done so within six months.
  - To evaluate patients' and healthcare professionals views of the workability and acceptability intervention and self administration service three months following implementation.

Once SMART objectives have been specified, you are then in a position to identify or devise suitable outcome measures for each. Think about each objective independently. How will it be addressed? In many cases, the literature will provide a useful source of possible approaches, methods and measures. If this is the case, incorporating established measures is often more robust than trying to devise your own. Otherwise, in a project that has a short timescale, you could end up spending most of the time developing and validating your methods and measures, leaving insufficient time for the main body of the work.

In planning a study it is common to overestimate the amount (number of objectives) that can be accomplished within a limited time. Thus, in addition to being detailed and clear, the objectives must be realistically achievable. If you have a series of objectives, you should ensure that they all can be addressed by the proposed methods. Attempting to meet too many objectives can be at the expense of achieving any of them properly.

A clear and precise statement of aims and objectives is important for:
- the selection of a suitable study design
- determining the most appropriate approach and methods so that all objectives are effectively addressed
- development of the instruments: in particular ensuring that all the necessary information is gathered (with attention to its completeness, reliability and validity), while avoiding the collection of unnecessary data (which lengthens questionnaires or interviews and is inefficient)
- specifying a framework and procedures for analysis.

Pilot studies

The aim of a pilot study is to ensure that the methods of the study are workable and acceptable for all participants, that the data will be sufficient and of adequate quality to achieve the study objectives. Many projects require some pilot work to be undertaken prior to commencement of the main study. This is because before you embark on the main study you want to check for any potential problems and if necessary make improvements. You may undertake a small amount of focused pilot work to check on particular aspects of the methods. For example, you may ask a few people to respond to a questionnaire to check the questions make sense to them. A true pilot study is a small version of a larger study, using the same population, methods and procedures. Sometimes, a student project comprises a pilot study prior to the development of a protocol for a much larger project. Pilot studies, in terms of their design and purpose are discussed in more detail in **Chapter 9**.

Research and ethics

Formal ethics approval is required for all healthcare research involving human participants. In the UK there are some exceptions to this, in that projects that are considered audits or service evaluations are viewed as an essential part of service delivery and not research. However, in these cases other permissions e.g. to comply with local research and development or audit procedures may be required. These local procedures are usually less complex than obtaining formal research ethics committee approval and obtainable within a shorter time frame. Obtaining formal approval from research ethics committees can be a lengthy process. If this is required, it needs to be obtained prior to the commencement of project. Thus, the involvement of students working on a 3-6 month project in this process will often be very limited. However, an understanding of research ethics is crucial to an appreciation of the research process. Moreover, whether or not you have been involved in an application to a formal body for ethical approval you should be able to demonstrate an understanding of the principles and approaches of ethical review.

Whether or not formal approval from a research ethics committee is required, all projects raise ethical dilemmas. If you are working on a project that does not require a formal application, you should still apply a systematic approach to identifying and addressing any potential ethical issues. Similarly, even if you believe your study does not present controversial ethical dilemmas you need to justify this viewpoint, again by applying a systematic approach to defending this position.

Ethical issues can be wide ranging. Therefore, in reviewing research ethics it can be helpful to draw on an established framework. One approach that can be applied is the Foster framework.[1] This comprises three sets of questions that enable you to conduct an ethical appraisal from three different perspectives (*Box 3.3*). This framework highlights, firstly, the goals of the research, whether these are worthy and likely to be achieved by the project; secondly, your duty as a researcher to ensure that what you are asking of organisations or participants is reasonable and justified; and thirdly, the rights of the participants, in particular that these are respected. These three perspectives and the questions you might ask yourself in relation to each are discussed below. However, many of these may not apply to a particular study, conversely there may be other issues that are not included.

Box 3.3: The three perspectives of the Foster framework[1] in ethical review

1. The goal-based perspective: Are the aims of the project worthy? Are they likely to be achieved by this work?
2. The duty-based perspective: Is what you are asking of organisations and/or participants reasonable and justified?
3. The rights-based perspective: Are the rights of the participants being respected?

---

1.   Foster C. *The Ethics of Research on Humans*. Cambridge: Cambridge University Press, 2001.

Goal-based questions

When approving a study, an ethics committee will want to be satisfied of the ultimate value of the project, i.e. that it is worth doing. If it is not original or important, or it does not appear that it will be carried out in a scientific manner, it may be considered unethical to devote time and resources. It should be clear that research that requires the dedicated funding, the time of health professionals, and/or may be a burden for potential participants, will ultimately be of value. Questions you might ask yourself from a goals' perspective are:

- Why is this study important?
- Is this the best way to address this research question?
- To what extent will the findings be representative and accurate?
- Are the anticipated findings likely to be relevant to the real needs of patients, health professionals and/or institutions, etc.?

Thus, in any application for ethical review, it is important to ensure that the relevance of the work, the expected value of the findings and the scientific validity of the project are clear and justified. In any application, it should not be left to committee members to wonder about the value of the work. Other general issues to consider may be provision for involvement of representatives of the study population, attention to the special needs of particular groups, or people who speak other languages.

Your duty to prospective participants

Once the overall value of the project has been considered, you could then think about the methods and procedures of the study from the perspective of those people who will be involved. As a researcher you have a duty to your participants to make sure that you are not making unreasonable demands. Questions to ask from a duty-based perspective may be:

- What are you asking people to do? Are these requests reasonable?
- Are you putting participants at unnecessary risk or inconvenience?
- Are the special needs of any particular groups identified and addressed?

If the work involves older people, children, or people who are sick or have other specific needs, guidance should be sought about additional considerations to safeguard their interests and rights. However worthy the goals of the study are, the dignity, rights, safety and well-being of participants are paramount.

In an ethical review, all aspects of the work should be critically considered so that potential concerns can be identified and addressed. For example, with regard to specific proposals for recruitment and data collection in a pharmacy practice project, you may consider the following:

- Are the procedures intrusive or too demanding? Are you expecting too much? Could the methods be modified?
- Does an interview schedule include sensitive questions or explore

topics that could be upsetting? If so, are you (and others involved in data collection) equipped to manage these situations? Is appropriate guidance provided?

- Could the questions uncover concerns about the quality of care that a patient is receiving? If so, how will this be handled?
- Could any of the questioning or observational procedures cause embarrassment? Will people be afforded sufficient privacy?
- Could there be security concerns with regard to interviews conducted in people's own homes? If so, can you ensure that the interviewee is provided with information to identify the researcher in advance? The safety of the researchers must also be considered.
- If you are employing others to assist with the data collection, how will you ensure that the study protocol will be closely followed by all?
- What are you going to do with the information you collect?
- What happens if someone complains or something goes wrong?

Respecting the rights of participants

A rights-based appraisal is the final perspective. All projects should be conducted in such a way that the rights of potential participants are respected. Key features of this perspective are:

- full information
- genuine choice regarding participation
- confidentiality of data.

Informed consent is central to research ethics. Participants should be fully informed as to what their participation will involve and how the data will be used, and should have opportunities to ask questions. Without this they will not be in a position to make an informed decision on whether or not to take part. Deception on any of these points will not allow informed consent and will therefore be deemed unethical. Participants must feel free to make a choice and they should have time to consider their decision. They should also be assured that they are free to opt out at any time should they change their mind and that this would not affect their care or rights in any way.

Participants' rights to confidentiality must also be respected. Researchers will not have access to health or personal information of participants before obtaining their informed consent. Even once informed consent has been obtained, researchers must only access information for the purpose of the research project. Safeguards to ensure the confidentiality of data must be in place, e.g. consent forms with participants' names should be stored separately from the data, and only the members of the research team should have access to identity codes on questionnaires or other data collection documents. Identity codes should be unique for the study, not numbers or codes that are used for other purposes e.g. NHS numbers that may allow the participant to be identified. All data should be anonymised, names being omitted during the transcribing process.

Information leaflets should be prepared, possibly being distributed with letters inviting individuals to participate. These should explain to potential participants the purposes of the study, who is organising, funding and responsible for the work, and how and why particular people have been chosen to take part. Details of study procedures should be provided so that it is clear to people what will happen should they agree to take part. Potential participants should also be informed that their participation is voluntary, they are free to withdraw at any time, and all information will be kept strictly confidential and anonymised so that no one is identifiable in the results. Contact details should be provided so that people are able to seek further information. Information about transparency of the processing of personal data should be included in the information leaflet for UK studies. General data protection regulations apply to all personal data being processed in the UK. Data is considered to be personal if it is identifiable or where the participant can be identified in combination with other data being held. Researchers need to provide transparency information about the legal basis and other details of processing such data. For pharmacy projects, the legal basis is likely to be that it is a task in the public interest. Participants should be informed on who will have access to their personal data and what they will use it for.

A proforma information sheet produced by the ethics committee may be suitable for adaptation for the study.

Arrangements should be put in place to ensure all potential participants can access the information including those with a disability or for whom English is not their first language.

Written consent is generally required for all studies and must be obtained before the start of any data collection. The consent form often comprises a series of statements relating to the information and procedures of the project, with a space against each statement for participants to initial to indicate their understanding and/or consent. The form should be dated and signed by the participant and sometimes also by the person taking the consent. A check list of questions for you to consider might include:

- Is an information leaflet supplied that conforms to accepted guidelines?
- Is there an opportunity to ask questions?
- What steps will you take to ensure confidentiality/ anonymity e.g. with data protection legislation and general data protection regulation?
- Are potential participants free to make their own decision e.g. time to decide, no incentives, possible concerns about consequences or taking/ not taking part or feelings of obligation?

Irrespective of external requirements for ethical review, many of the considerations above may apply. Therefore, you should always be mindful of your duties and responsibilities and observe high ethical standards in the conduct of a project.

When formal ethical approval is required, data collection for a study cannot proceed until it has been obtained. Although limited preliminary fieldwork (e.g. informal discussions with colleagues) may be undertaken before seeking ethical approval, formal pilot work with potential research participants does not occur until approval is obtained. Thus, the timing of seeking ethical approval is important, as the process can be lengthy. It is important to plan ahead, to find out the exact requirements for the applications to these bodies and to prepare the documentation as soon as possible.

An application to a research ethics committee will generally include all documentation relating to the study: a protocol describing the aims and objectives, all methods and procedures, including those to ensure the validity of data, will be required. Copies of the instruments (e.g. questionnaires, interview schedules, any other data collection forms), information leaflets, consent forms, letters of recruitment, other documentation, etc. should also be included.

Conclusion

The preparatory stages of any project are vital to its ultimate success. A project in a limited time frame must be carefully planned to ensure that the aims and objectives are worthwhile and achievable. The methods must be an acceptable, feasible and effective means of obtaining sufficient and quality data. The methodology and operation of a project is often guided by a protocol, which should provide sufficient detail to enable identification and discussion of potential ethical issues that the project presents. It is the researcher's responsibility to ensure that necessary permissions are obtained and that in the execution of the study they operate ethically and professionally throughout.

Questions

1. What is project protocol?

How might these objectives be made smarter?

2. To identify the number of medication prescribing errors on wards.

3. To identify how many patients switched from natalizumab to fingolimod.

4. When is formal research ethics committee approval required in the UK? (Select all that apply)
   A: For all healthcare research involving human subjects
   B: For all healthcare research involving changes to treatment
   C: For all research involving invasive procedures
   D: For all service evaluations involving human subjects
   E: For all audits involving human subjects

You are on a local ethics committee at your hospital. Look at the scenarios below. What ethical issues may arise? How could the investigators be asked to address these issues?

5. Some researchers need to collect data about a patients' antibiotic treatment. They state that on the data collection form they will record the patients' initials.

6. Some researchers need to collect data on a rare condition at a hospital trust. They state that they will anonymise the patients identified by giving them each a numerical ID.

7. A team of healthcare professionals want to audit the behaviour of healthcare professionals on a ward to see how well they treat patients at risk of nutritional difficulties. However, they do not want them to change their behaviour as a result of observing them. They have decided to tell the healthcare professionals that they are observing them for a different reason.

You are carrying out a project at your hospital. The following situations arise. What ethical issues are involved? How could you address them?

8. You are looking at some data on a database about hospital patients. Your friend knows someone who is one of the hospital wards and wants to find out how she is. She asks you if you can have a look at her notes while you are logged into the system.

9. You are conducting an audit on safe prescribing practices. While you are looking at patient data you notice a mistake that may be harmful to a patient if it is not corrected.

10. You are inviting a participant to take part in your study. You give them the information leaflet to read but they are partially sighted and are having some difficulties reading it.

CHAPTER 4

Time management and working with others

Effective organisation and time management is an essential component of successful pharmacy projects. As identified in **Chapter 2** there are many stages to a project and you need to plan when you will carry out each of them in order to finish your project on time. In pharmacy practice projects there are likely to be some quieter periods, for example while you are waiting for local approvals. Planning for these and identifying other tasks that can be done during these less busy periods will help you make more effective use of your time.

In the early stages of the work, and with the help of your supervisor, you should come up with a feasible time plan covering the duration of the project. This will be helpful in enabling you to form an overview of the entire project. It will require identifying the different tasks involved and estimating how long each will take.

Researchers are often overambitious regarding what can be achieved within a limited period. The time taken for some tasks is commonly underestimated - it is important to be realistic. In particular, the preparation of applications to ethics committees and obtaining approval, recruitment of participants, waiting for return of completed questionnaires and arranging interviews to suit the availability of others can be lengthy tasks over which you have only limited control. Following up non-responders to questionnaires, transcribing audio-recorded data, checking data for accuracy and coding and analysing qualitative data sets can be very time-consuming. Preparing a Gantt chart and specifying milestones are common aids to time management of a project.

A Gantt chart

A Gantt chart (*Figure 4.1*) is often used as an aid to project planning and to ensure timely completion. A Gantt chart includes all the activities to be undertaken in the project in detail, in the order in which they are expected to commence, and plots out the time that will be allocated to each. Many activities will overlap and can operate concurrently. For example, it would be sensible to commence the literature review whilst waiting for permission to commence fieldwork. If time permits, the methods sections of the project report can be written up whilst data collection is ongoing.

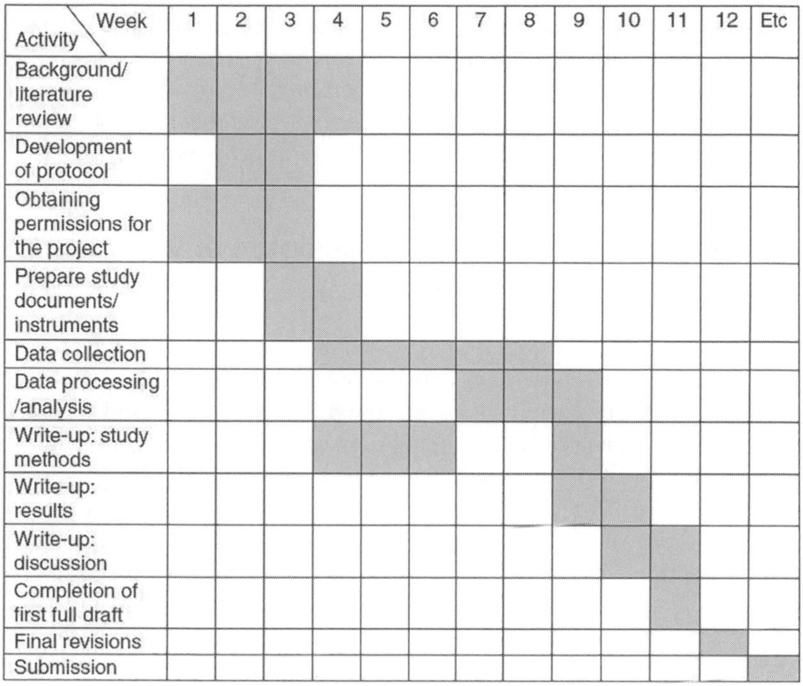

Activity \ Week	1	2	3	4	5	6	7	8	9	10	11	12	Etc
Background/ literature review	▓	▓	▓										
Development of protocol		▓	▓										
Obtaining permissions for the project	▓	▓	▓										
Prepare study documents/ instruments			▓										
Data collection				▓	▓	▓	▓						
Data processing /analysis						▓	▓	▓					
Write-up: study methods				▓	▓	▓			▓				
Write-up: results									▓	▓			
Write-up: discussion										▓	▓		
Completion of first full draft											▓		
Final revisions												▓	
Submission													▓

Figure 4.1: *An example of a Gantt chart*

Milestones

Project milestones are dates by which specific activities of the project are to be achieved. These should be listed out as 'activity' with a date. Typical milestones might be:

- Completion of full draft of literature review (and submission to supervisor)
- Final version of protocol, preparation of a Gantt chart
- Start and/or completion of data collection
- Completion of specified sections of project write-up
- Submission of final project report

Milestones should be discussed and agreed with your supervisor - this will help ensure they are realistic. It is worth considering that many tasks are likely to take longer than you might initially expect. For example, you may need to work up several drafts of the protocol before agreeing this with your supervisor and commencing data collection. Recruitment is often the process which runs slower than expected. It is sensible to identify some contingency plans, for example by allowing additional time for the recruitment stage and/or for the potential use of other sources of data. The times at which you will submit work to your supervisors should be agreed and recorded on your Gantt chart. This will also enable the timing of submission of your work for comment to take account of their other commitments. The most appropriate points at which to meet your supervisor may also be when you anticipate reaching a milestone or embarking on a new aspect of the project, thus progress can be reviewed and subsequent stages can be discussed.

Working with others in a professional environment

Working with supervisors

During your project you will need to work closely with your supervisor(s). It is important that you develop a professional approach, such as attending meetings punctually, keeping them informed of your progress and sending work when agreed. Your supervisors are there to guide you but it is ultimately your project and you must take ownership of it. It is your responsibility to arrange meetings with your supervisor. Giving thought to what you want to achieve in each meeting, taking effective meeting notes, including action points and sharing them with your supervisor(s) can be helpful. You may have more than one supervisor for your project, and you need to collaborate with both of them and ensure they are both kept fully informed of all decisions relating to your project. Copying both supervisors into all communications can be an effective strategy for this.

Working with research participants

People who participate in your study are often doing this out of good will. They will almost invariably have competing demands on their time, will usually derive no direct benefit and will agree to take part because they can see that the work may be of some future value. If you are a student they may see this value as limited to educational objectives. People will often be agreeable only if they can see that the work is relevant to some aspect of service development or patient care, carefully planned and professionally conducted, and that their rights are being observed. Although many studies depend on the goodwill of individuals, sometimes a nominal payment is made to participants in recognition of their time, expertise and to reimburse any expenses.

In conducting your project, attention should be paid to maintaining a professional approach: good time keeping, appropriate self-presentation, adherence to agreed study procedures and ensuring that the involvement of others is straightforward and procedures result in minimum inconvenience. As the researcher you must be willing to accommodate the commitments of participants (e.g. by arranging interviews at their convenience) and not expect them to fall in line. Forethought in ensuring that the procedures are workable in each setting will assist in the smooth operation and acceptability of the project, e.g. make sure that any need for access to a computer, powerpoints, other facilities or documents will not hinder the work of staff, maintain a supply of spare batteries for recording equipment, etc. Throughout the work, it is the student who should 'do the running' and fit around the priorities and commitments of others, and not vice versa. An unprofessional approach could both jeopardise your work and discourage individuals from participating in future studies.

Records should be maintained of all meetings that you have. These may be discussions with key practitioners or representatives of other stakeholders in the planning of your work. You should keep notes of the advice you receive and how this influenced your ideas for the study, and/or the documents, procedures and methods. You can then acknowledge this input as 'personal communication' in your final report.

You should also keep careful records of all contacts with potential participants (including personal, telephone, email, social media, and post). It is very easy to forget who asked for more information, declined to participate, asked you to phone them back at a later date, were on holiday, etc. Some of this information may enable you to comment on the ease of setting up the study, acceptability of the methods and how in future they might be improved. Notes should be made of any reasons given for non-response. Details of any difficulties experienced in the execution of the study may be helpful in assessments of validity and any shortcomings in the study.

Having taken part in a study, participants may like to be informed of the findings. It is good practice, after completion of the work, to send a letter of thanks and offer a summary of the findings to everyone who was involved. If the work is published, a copy of the paper can be sent when this becomes available. However, publication is generally a protracted process, usually at least one, and sometimes more than two years from data collection. Participants should be informed of the anticipated duration of the study and when to expect information about the findings. A list of names and addresses of all participants and others who have assisted in the work or expressed an interest should be maintained and the information about the findings forwarded as soon as possible.

Working with others and group projects

Pharmacy practice projects are almost invariably collaborative. At the very least, you are likely to require the cooperation of others during the data collection e.g. as respondents to questionnaires, interviewees or hosts who agree to the presence of a student on their premises. Projects in health services research are commonly interdisciplinary and the contributions of people from different backgrounds and with particular skills and experience can be invaluable in ensuring that different perspectives are taken into account. There is an increasing emphasis on working with members of the public and in ensuring that this involvement is meaningful rather than tokenistic. This is discussed in more detail in **Chapter 5** where we give a step-by-step guide to how to bring a high level of patient and public involvement to your project.

When working with others it is important to be clear from the start what the respective role and responsibilities of each person will be. For some projects, the level of involvement of different individuals will vary e.g. some people may take responsibility for particular tasks or contribute expertise at a certain stage of the work. In other projects a group may work as a team, in which the levels of commitment of all members are expected to be similar and the responsibilities for all stages of the work are shared.

Some group projects fall naturally into a number of discrete parts. If this is so, each member of the team can take responsibility for one part, working more or less independently on this, albeit within an agreed broad framework. In other cases, the team as a whole may be responsible for planning a project, developing a protocol, data collection, processing and analysis and writing the final report. A team approach can confer a number of advantages. Ideas and expertise can be pooled and the objectives might be more ambitious e.g. it may provide an opportunity to address a topic from a wider range of perspectives. It may be possible to extend sampling over a larger number of locations or to different groups of respondents. These features may enhance the relevance, generalisability and value of the work.

Working in a team requires careful preparation. It is usually helpful if the team elects a chairperson (this role can rotate around the group members) – it generally leads to more productive meetings. Each meeting should have an agenda. The chairperson has responsibility for ensuring that all items are addressed. Another group member should be responsible for taking notes of the decisions made and the division of work. At the end of every meeting all group members should agree and be clear about the tasks that they are to undertake. If the project is to be successful, cooperation in planning, commitment to the group effort and adherence to agreed study protocols are essential. Unilateral decisions on the approach and methods by individuals regarding separate components of the project may undermine its integrity as a whole.

If a number of people are involved in collecting data for a project, you will also want to have systems in place for everyone to follow. This will help make sure that everyone operates in a similar way and the data collected by each person are comparable. In meetings, you may want to share experiences in conducting the work so you can identify any inconsistencies or problems that arise. As for all projects, the earlier problems are identified the better. Once data collection has progressed remedial action is difficult. Early recognition of, and attention to, problems will greatly enhance the accuracy, completeness and usefulness of the data.

Conclusion

Devising a realistic time plan in the early stages will increase the chances of timely operation and completion of the project. Careful forethought is required recognising the likely times required for arranging meetings, obtaining permissions to undertake the work, accessing and collecting data. Throughout the duration of the project, the activities should be planned and paced so there is sufficient time for all stages right through to the writing up and final presentation. Many projects in a professional setting depend on the cooperation of others. Early discussions will ensure that project goals, methods and timescales are realistic from all perspectives.

Questions

1. **Choose the statement that you agree with the most. In a group project, in order to ensure consistent, reliable outcomes:**

   A: There must never be any deviation from the protocol

   B: Any deviation from the protocol that is proposed should be discussed and addressed by the full team

   C: Some deviation without discussion is acceptable

   D: Researchers in a group should be able to make decisions regarding adherence to the protocol independently

2. **List typical milestones in a pharmacy practice project.**

3. **How can you plan ahead to ensure that your project will be completed on time?**

4. **What are the potential uncertainties that could prevent the timely completion of your project and how might they be addressed?**

5. **Identifying the stakeholders you will need to engage with during your project, outlining the potential contribution of each.**

CHAPTER 5

Patient and public involvement

LEARNING OBJECTIVES

Upon completion of this chapter you should be able to:

- explain the difference between patient and public participation, engagement and involvement
- describe different levels of patient and public involvement
- describe the roles which patient and public representatives can have in pharmacy practice projects
- develop terms of partnership between patient and public representatives and researchers
- identify the challenges that may occur in engaging with patient and public representatives and how these might be mitigated.

Patient and public involvement in service evaluations and research is growing. Funding bodies are increasingly asking about arrangements for patient and public involvement before funding research. It is recognised that studies are more likely to be tailored to the needs of patients and members of the public if patients and the public are involved in planning, delivering and monitoring them. Such involvement can increase the quality of studies and improve their translation into practice. In addition, it is democratic and transparent to involve people who are affected by research in the planning of it, particularly if the research is publicly funded.

Patient and public involvement differs from participation and engagement. Participation refers to taking part in research as a subject or participant, for example taking part in a randomised controlled trial, or completing a questionnaire or interview. Engagement refers to activities relating to acquiring knowledge of studies and sharing findings e.g. attending open days or festivals to find out more about research that is taking place. In contrast, involvement refers to building partnerships with researchers and influencing what studies are done, how they are done and what happens to the findings. The focus in this chapter is on involvement. There has been increasing emphasis on ensuring that patients and members of the public are involved in studies as true partners, rather than being on the margins to fulfil the requirements of a funding body. Terms that are increasingly being used are co-production and co-design, where healthcare professionals and members of the public come together as equals to design a service/study together.

This chapter has been written in collaboration with seven patient and public involvement representatives who have been involved in research projects and includes quotations from them.

Why do patients and members of the public become involved in research?

Patients and members of the public may become involved in research for many reasons. It may be to champion a particular cause or a more general interest e.g. to 'keep the brain cells working and continue to be helpful to others following retirement.' Many people get involved for the public good, to show tangible gratitude for healthcare services they have received, i.e. 'to put something back into the system'. Sometimes patients and members of the public can be motivated by previous experiences they have had as a patient or in a previous career, which they feel allows them to contribute.

Levels of patient and public involvement

Patient and public involvement takes place on many levels ranging from minimal to consultation, to collaboration, to patient- and public-led. Consultation refers to one-off events where patient and public representatives are asked to give their opinions. For example, they might be asked to participate in a focus group to decide on priorities for a particular research area, or they might be asked their opinion of a patient information leaflet.

Collaboration refers to ongoing partnership throughout a project; 'end-to-end lay engagement'. In collaborative projects, participants will be involved throughout a project, rather than at a specific point in time. They will develop ongoing partnerships with the researchers, be part of the research team or advisory group and contribute at all stages. Collaboration is the minimum level regarded as being satisfactory by many patient and public representatives.

Finally, patient- and public-led projects will be run by patient and public representatives who will ask the researchers for their input. Patients may have an initial idea for a research project and will then work with researchers to deliver it. This is rare and it is more common for researchers and patient and public representatives to work collaboratively together.

As well as these more formal definitions, different levels of involvement may also be derived from the experience of patient and public representatives. This is how one patient and public representative who had been involved in many projects described the different levels of involvement he had experienced:

- Level 1 – 'Tick box (tending towards tokenism)'
- Level 2 – 'Commitment by the researchers to patient and public involvement, but only partial cultural sign-up (brave attempt but don't entirely get it)'
- Level 3 – 'All singing all dancing (regular communication flows, clear desire to listen to external views and to consider making changes in the light of them, making PPI volunteers feel part of the team)'

Below is a quote from a patient and public representative who felt that the third level had been reached in a project she had been working on, and that the researchers and patient and public involvement representatives had worked synergistically:

'What was very important is that everyone's contribution could be inserted in a very natural way; it wasn't someone providing a contribution in isolation – like in a tunnel, which sometimes can happen. It was basically a very rich mosaic of contribution and views all meshing together to provide a very, very rich outcome.'

Roles that patient and public representatives have in pharmacy practice projects

In general, patient and public representatives prefer to be involved in projects at the earliest stage possible as it gives them maximum opportunity to shape the project, and a sense of ownership within it. In any case, patient and public involvement will need to be planned early in order to budget for it.

One role for patient and public representatives is in *helping to decide what projects are carried out*. Patient and public representatives can be involved in deciding on research priorities generally and/or developing specific proposals. They are increasingly co-applicants on grant applications.

Other roles evolve around individual projects. A minimal role which patient and public representatives would generally have in a project would be to *input into the patient-facing materials and plain English summaries*. The former includes patient information leaflets, consent forms, questionnaires, interview schedules and topic guides. Patient and public representatives can either comment on materials first produced by researchers, or be involved in developing the materials.

Patient and public representatives often have a role in the *management and monitoring of projects*. They may be part of the advisory or steering group for projects. Having a patient and public co-chair, or chair of such a group, can increase partnership and help even out any power imbalances in the group. The advisory group can receive regular progress reports detailing the project activities that have taken place, those planned, and any challenges that have arisen. Reports may provide information about whether or not the project is on target and any actions that the advisory group members can take to input into the study.

A relatively rarer, but growing, role is for patient and public members to take part in *conducting the research*. This may include taking part in data collection e.g. conducting interviews or carrying out observations either on their own or together with researchers. For example, patient and public representatives may observe consultations between pharmacists and patients and give their perspective on these. Patient and public representatives may also *take part in data analysis*, either by suggesting analysis to be carried out or actively carrying out analysis. For example, they may review a sample of interview transcripts and openly code them to identify key themes in the data. These may then be compared and integrated with the themes identified by researchers. There is room to give patient and public representatives the choice of the extent to which they wish to be involved in data collection and analysis and how. For example, they might be asked how many consultations they would like to observe, how many interviews they would like to analyse, and/or whether they would like to use a framework, or do open coding analysis.

Patient and public representatives can also have a key role in the *dissemination of findings and increasing impact*. This may be through suggesting routes for publication, directly disseminating findings through their networks, or developing materials for dissemination, particularly those aimed at patients, carers and members of the public. Examples may include leaflets, infographics and videos. Most research reports now include a lay summary, which patient and public representatives can contribute to, as a minimum. Roles may extend to being authors on papers if they meet authorship criteria or co-presenting project findings at meetings, seminars and conferences.

The above is not an exhaustive list. Patients and members of the public can be involved at any stage of the project, even those that may not seem obvious. For example, they have been involved in recruiting participants for a study and in reviewing the key literature identified by a research team and providing their perspectives on its relevance to an ongoing project.

Recruiting patient and public representatives
When recruiting patient and public representatives it is important to consider what roles you are expecting them to have in a project and the level of involvement. As noted in the previous section, there are a large number of potential roles which patient and public representatives can have in projects. You need to be clear about what you are asking them to do, how much time it is likely to take up, and expenses and honorarium that they will receive.

Much the same as in other recruitment process, you will then need to think about who you need and why. You need to consider the type of person who would be best to fulfil the roles you have identified. For example, are you looking for people with a specific condition, taking particular types of medication, or having had certain types of experiences? Are you looking for people who have been involved in research projects before or those who may be 'a fresh pair of eyes'? Both have their advantages and disadvantages. Those who have worked with researchers before will have a good understanding of the processes involved, which may help optimise their contributions. They may also be able to provide innovative insights from cross-pollination with other projects they may be involved in. However, there is also a danger of developing 'patient and public experts' who may no longer completely represent the general patient and public population. It can often be good to have a mixture of people with different backgrounds working on a project. Each patient and public representative can bring their own experiences to the table e.g. of being a patient, being a carer, working with consumers, working with policymakers, etc.

Once you have identified who you need to recruit, the next stage is to think about sources of potential partners. Universities and healthcare organisations will sometimes have their own networks of patient and public representatives who can be invited to participate. These representatives will probably have some experience of research involvement. Patient and public representatives may also be recruited from patient charities and support groups. These patients will probably have experience of a particular condition but may not have been involved in research before. Social media may be used to advertise opportunities. In addition, 'People in Research' is a website that has been set up in order to help members of the public who would like to get involved in research find opportunities and researchers to find members of the public to contribute to their research (*www.peopleinresearch.org*). Researchers can post opportunities here.

Recruitment processes can be similar to recruitment to any other role; setting selection criteria, creating an application form, inviting applications and arranging to meet with potential partners.

Developing terms of partnership with patient and public representatives

It is good practice to discuss, agree and clearly set out partnership terms with patient and public representatives in order to manage everyone's expectations and avoid misunderstandings. The UK organisation INVOLVE (*www.involve.org.uk*) recommends developing role descriptions for patient and public representatives. These should set out:

- the scope of involvement including what may have already been agreed and does not have room for change; for example, aspects of the project that have already been agreed with the funding body
- the activities that patient and public representatives would be expected to be involved in during the course of a study; for example how many meetings they would need to attend, how much preparation they would need to do for these meetings, and any other activities they would be involved in such as reviewing documents, etc.
- the responsibilities of the project team towards their patient and public representatives. This should include payments that they will receive, and other benefits such as provision of refreshments at meetings and training opportunities. Ideally, patient and public representatives should be asked what training needs they have, their preferences, and the way they would like to receive training. A research buddy scheme may also be offered where a patient and public representative buddies with a researcher during the project. When thinking about training, a balance needs to be struck between helping patient and public representatives to develop skills needed, while also ensuring that their own unique contribution as patient and public representatives is not compromised
- the methods by which patient and public representatives will be given feedback on how their input has been incorporated into the study. Having

spent considerable time and energy inputting they like to know what value they have added.

Some of these aspects will need to be decided before recruitment, so that applicants are informed about what they might be taking on. However, there should also be flexibility to develop these throughout a project in response to patient and public representatives' needs, preferences and experiences. This is crucial to forming equal partnerships and helping patient and public representatives fully integrate into the team.

Setting up the first project meeting

Following recruitment, the next stage will be to set up the first meeting. Ideally, patients and public representatives should be involved in setting the date to ensure it is convenient for them. For example, some potential dates could be identified and participants be offered the opportunity to vote for a specific date. Prior to the meeting, it is also important to invite participants to inform you of any specific needs they have and discuss how these can be met. In the fortnight before the meeting, you will then need to send out a meeting agenda together with clear directions on how to reach the venue.

Holding the first project meeting

During the first meeting you may wish to spend some time on introductions to help the group start to come together. You may also wish to facilitate this by asking advisory group members to create a short paragraph about themselves that you circulate before the meeting. Following introductions, you may wish to give an overview of the project, the timescales and your thoughts on their involvement. While role descriptions will have been created prior to the recruitment process, this is an opportunity to discuss the way the collaboration will work in more detail and ensure that patient and public representatives are part of the process of creating them. Examples of details that are good to discuss are training needs, specific requirements, chairing of meetings, location and timing of meetings and preferences for receipt of documents. At this stage you will need to go through any administrative procedures that are relevant, for example how patient and public representatives can claim payments for their involvement and when they can expect to receive these payments. Finally, you will probably have specific issues relating to your project that you would like to discuss at this meeting.

Challenges that may arise with patient and public involvement and how to mitigate these

Misunderstandings and breakdowns in communication can sometimes occur between patient and public representatives and researchers. The process of patient and public involvement in research involves the coming together of three different cultures: the patient and public culture, the healthcare professional culture and the research culture. Sometimes things that seem obvious to one party may not be as obvious to another. For example, there may be different assumptions around issues of informed consent, confidentiality and engaging with social media. While patient and public representatives will have their own ethical and moral principles that they will follow, these will not always match the ethical codes of researchers. An example would be making a decision that collecting data from interesting cases, potentially of great value in informing future practice, overrides the requirement to obtain informed consent. The main way to mitigate these is through very clear and precise communication at all times. Patient and public representatives will only know that you would like something kept confidential or out of social media if you tell them.

It can also be helpful to manage expectations. Patient and public representatives will often be busy people with several work, family or volunteering commitments. It is always preferable to give them advance notice of when you will need their input and allow them sufficient time to respond to requests for feedback wherever possible. Of course, projects are not always predictable and situations may arise where you need unplanned input. For example, you may need the review of a long document very quickly. In that case, it would be good practice to explain to patient and public representatives why you need the feedback so quickly, to ask them to perhaps focus on specific parts where their input would be most valuable and to say you understand if they are not able to comment.

Patient and public representatives who are involved in your project may have chronic conditions which may affect their level of involvement at times. For example, they may have a flare-up of a physical or mental health condition. They may also be caring for someone and need to fit their involvement around the needs of the care recipient. Again, clear communication at the start is vital to managing this process. Finding out their needs, offering flexibility, allowing them to dial-in to meetings, and being understanding if they need to step back for a while are all vital in managing this process. Having a small team of patient and public representatives will help ensure there is continuous involvement, even at times when some representatives need to step back.

Sometimes patient and public representatives may come with strong views, be quite dominant in meetings, and/or be interested in areas not specifically relevant to the project. A good first step would be to try and manage this within the meetings. It is important to structure the meeting so that patient and public representatives can contribute what they feel is important, while not allowing discussions that are not directly relevant to take over the meeting. One strategy may be to agree the agenda beforehand with the patient and public representatives, including the time that will be devoted to each item. However, if this is not possible or not working, an alternative solution may be to set up a separate individual meeting to discuss their concerns and agree a way forward.

Both patient and public representatives and researchers may experience negative emotions during the course of a project. For example, patient and public representatives have reported sometimes feeling overwhelmed if they felt underprepared, that they had a lack of knowledge, or that the project was moving beyond their skill set. Using the buddy system described above, checking in regularly with patient and public representatives during a study, avoiding the use of jargon, and ensuring that researchers' expertise is not allowed to dominate will all help mitigate against this. Patient and public representatives can also sometimes become distressed when hearing about, or seeing others' experiences, particularly if these open up emotions within them that have been previously buried. It is important to be aware of this, anticipate where possible, and support patient and public representatives accordingly. Researchers may experience upset and anxiety if they feel criticised by patient and public representatives, or feel under threat from them bringing their own perspectives, which may be different from those of researchers. It is important to recognise that the strength of patient and public representatives' involvement is in the different viewpoints that this brings, that their perspectives can conflict with those of researchers, and that working to join researchers' and patient and public viewpoints together as one is where the most added value from patient/public partnerships comes.

Monitoring and reporting on impact of patient and public involvement

It is good practice to capture the impact of patient and public involvement in projects. This is important for understanding your findings and informing future practice, both for those involved in the project and other researchers. Try to involve patient and public representatives in planning how their input will be evaluated as well as in the actual evaluation of their impact and their experiences of involvement.

Conclusion

In summary, patient and public representatives can potentially bring a huge amount to a project and be involved at every stage. To maximise this potential it is important to keep in dialogue at all times, ask about their experiences, needs and preferences, and be open to their perspectives.

Questions

1. **Which of the following activities might patient and public representatives contribute to? (Select all that apply)**
   A: Deciding what research to carry out
   B: Literature review
   C: Reviewing a patient information leaflet
   D: Recruiting participants to a study
   E: Interviewing participants
   F: Analysing data
   G: Monitoring progress
   H: Disseminating project findings

2. **Explain the differences between consultation, collaboration and patient- and public-led involvement.**

3. **How can researchers ensure that patient and public representatives feel part of the team?**

4. **Name three challenges that may occur when working with members of the public, and what you would do to mitigate them.**

5. **Explain how you think patient and public involvement representatives could contribute to your project.**

CHAPTER 6

For supervisors

LEARNING OBJECTIVES

Upon completion of this chapter you should be able to:

- identify the value of pharmacy practice projects to students and supervisors
- identify the key roles that practice-based supervisors have in pharmacy practice projects
- identify strategies for working effectively with university-based supervisors
- identify strategies for assisting the student with time planning and project write-up
- develop a meeting schedule together with the student.

Practising pharmacists working in community and hospital settings are taking an increasing role in co-supervising projects with university supervisors. This can provide a huge range of opportunities for students to spend an extended period in a professional setting and to experience audit, service evaluation and research integrated into every day practice, rather than being limited to academic settings. Practice-based supervisors will generally have a great deal of professional expertise and knowledge of their clinical area that they can bring to the project. They may have a range of different experiences of research methods and of conducting and supervising pharmacy practice projects, with this being a new area to some. This chapter aims to provide guidance to supervisors in how to support students into carrying out a successful project.

Due to the great variety in the types of projects that students undertake, and the place of the research project in different university programmes, this chapter can only be viewed as a general guide. However, its content is based on the many requests for advice from new supervisors regarding the level and type of support that should be provided, the partnership with the university, and the extent to which students themselves should take responsibility for the work. Ideally, projects should meet the needs of both students and supervisors. Students, in the course of achieving their learning objectives, have the opportunity to be involved in original projects that are relevant and valuable to current service provision or research agendas. If the project is successful, supervisors will have assistance with a study that will support a wider research programme, and/or answer questions that are pertinent to their professional practice.

Types of project

There is huge variability in the types of project that students may be involved in. **Chapter 2** gives more information about the differences between research, service evaluation and audit to help identify which the student's project is, and the effect of this on the approvals required. This is important as there is unlikely to be sufficient time for a student to obtain full ethics approval during a study.

Some student projects form a component of a larger programme where there is limited opportunity to redefine the conceptual and methodological approach. Thus, students are participating in a study for which the objectives have already been defined and the methods decided. In evaluations or audits of professional practice or medicines use, the objectives may also be clear at the outset. Other projects, for example those intended to inform a new line of enquiry, may provide a greater opportunity for the student to influence the focus and course of the project: the actual research question may be decided following a review of the literature or once preliminary fieldwork has been undertaken. In some cases, the preliminary fieldwork may form the basis of the project.

A formal systematic literature review may or may not be required, depending on the university course regulations. However, the student should develop a strategy and procedures for identifying relevant literature so that they achieve an appreciation of the existing knowledge of the topic, lines of enquiry, current debates and viewpoints, and the relevance of the research question to policy, practice and/or patient care (*Box 6.1*). They should understand the literature well enough to build a case for why the current project is necessary. See **Chapter 8** for more information about conducting a literature review.

Projects will also differ in how the ownership, responsibilities and decision making are shared. This is inevitable. However, it is important that there is scope for students to assume a degree of ownership and responsibility which will require them to make some decisions regarding the operation of the data collection, the analysis and how to present and interpret their findings.

A diverse range of projects increases the opportunities for students to contribute to work that is timely. It enables students to appreciate the variety of research that is undertaken to advance pharmacy services and patient care. At the same time, students must achieve their learning objectives and adopt a scientific approach to produce findings that will be of value.

Box 6.1: A comprehensive literature review

- It is important to ensure that the work builds on existing theories or knowledge, and that it does not duplicate the work of others. It will help ensure that your work extends our knowledge or understanding in specific ways.
- It allows the identification of factors that have been found by other researchers to be important to the topic or issues under study, so they can be taken into account. These may relate to the setting of the research, particular structural or organisational factors or factors relevant to particular population groups.
- It enables the identification of the perspectives of different stakeholders, so that they can be considered.
- It assists in selecting the best methods for the study. There may be a number of ways of obtaining data relevant to the study objectives, all of which will have their strengths and weaknesses. Review of the methods used by others enables you to identify different options, together with their advantages and disadvantages, when planning your own study.

Role of practice-based supervisors

Support for the project will usually be shared with the university. Typically, the practice supervisor will identify the project area that would be valuable to their hospital or other practice setting, introduce the subject area to the student, provide guidance related to the clinical and practice area, help the student obtain local approvals required and oversee the day-to-day running of the project. They will also provide some direction for the literature review and methodology, supported also by the academic supervisor.

Role of university supervisors

Typically, the university supervisor will provide guidance for taking a systematic approach to the literature review, procedures for identifying relevant material, using databases and critically appraising different sources and types of evidence. They will also provide guidance on using robust research methods for the project and developing methods for the analysis. The university will usually also provide formal teaching on theoretical aspects of research methodology. This should provide an overview of different approaches and methods that are employed in research into service development, medicines use and professional practice.

Collaboration between the student, practice-based supervisor and university supervisor

To ensure a successful project, it is essential that the two supervisors and student work well together. As detailed above, the two supervisors will bring different expertise to the project and, if combined well, can provide a great deal of guidance and direction to the student. To effectively support the project, the academic supervisor will need to develop a good understanding of what the practice supervisor is hoping to gain from the project. This will feed greatly into the development of the aims and objectives. A potential pitfall of having two supervisors is that they may have different ideas and potentially provide conflicting advice to the student. This can be mitigated by encouraging the student to keep both supervisors informed of communications with the other. For example, they can be advised to copy both supervisors into email correspondence and to write and share notes of all meetings with both supervisors. Face-to-face meetings with both supervisors will often not be pragmatic due to the different locations in which they work; however, occasional telephone conferences may be helpful.

Time planning

For beneficial outcomes on both sides, some forward planning is essential. This increases the likelihood that the student's time will be used as effectively as possible, so that a useful project results. In making plans it may be helpful to think about the project from the perspectives of the student, the supervisor, as well as the course of the project itself.

Typically, undergraduate and masters projects are between 3 and 6 months' duration. They may be full-time or part-time (in that they run alongside other courses which require attendance by the student). In terms of planning this can be an important consideration. If the project is full-time, the work and commitment is more intense. Full-time projects have advantages in that students do not have to fit their project work around other commitments. However, any delays whilst waiting for approvals or other permissions, or arranging meetings with collaborators, can seriously impact on the remaining time available for research itself. For these projects, advance preparation can be particularly important if work is to start promptly. This will benefit the supervisor too, who ends up with a completed study rather than one which has just commenced. Part-time projects, if over a longer period, can often more easily accommodate the preparation and planning stages. However, once project work commences, the student may not have the flexibility of being able to meet with collaborators or collect data at times most convenient for others.

Assessments of the time required for each stage of project work should be realistic. It is easy to underestimate the time that may be required to obtain permissions to undertake the work and agreement of individuals to take part. A study can't commence until ethical clearance is obtained and key staff become available for discussion. Data collection may be paced by timing of clinic sessions, or recruitment of prospective participants, sending of reminders, ability to retrieve medical notes etc. It is also easy to be too optimistic about response rates and the time that individuals feel able to give to a project. Questions for supervisors to consider may be:

- Are there other people involved with whom meetings will be necessary?
- Will data collection only be possible at certain times?
- Will it be possible to collect sufficient data in the timescale of the project?
- Do special arrangements have to be made to accommodate the student or the operation of the study e.g. informing different staff members, access to computers or other equipment, space to conduct an interview or to take notes?
- Does documentation about the work need to be prepared in advance?
- Will some piloting be necessary?
- Will any committee approvals be required in advance e.g. audit, R&D, ethics?

Helping the student to prepare a timeline at the start can be very helpful. This should be a plan charting the tasks to be undertaken as part of the project against the calendar/time available. Estimates of the time required for all tasks should be made. (There is guidance for students in **Chapter 4** on time planning and preparation of a Gantt chart).

Dates of meetings must be set with the needs of the student, stages of the project and the commitments of the supervisor in mind. For most supervisors, project supervision needs to fit around other commitments. At times these other activities will have to take priority. Meeting dates should be arranged which, as far as possible, will be workable for the supervisor. Students must be aware that supervisors will have many other commitments and competing priorities around which project supervision has to be accommodated. From the point of view of the student, they should be informed of supervisors' availability and contact details. In the case of a need to change meetings or a prolonged absence, any necessary alternative plans should be put in place so that the students are able to continue with their work. Students will be anxious to use their time efficiently and effectively. Students, for their part, must appreciate the importance of taking responsibility for their project e.g. attending meetings with adequate preparation, submitting work on time and achieving project milestones as agreed.

At the start of the project the student will want to get going. If a supervisor cannot be around, a colleague or co-supervisor may be able to meet with the student to at least direct them on their background reading. Students may also need time at the start to familiarise themselves with the topic of the research, the environment in which they will be working and the methodology being used. Assisting them in preparing a realistic time plan at the start of their project will help to ensure effective and efficient use of the period available for project work.

All projects have busy and less busy times, over which the students and supervisors may have limited control. The quieter times are commonly towards the start of the project e.g. while waiting to meet with collaborators or for permissions to commence the work. Good project planning will ensure that quieter times are used productively. For many projects it is wise to undertake, and if possible complete, the background reading and literature work in the first few weeks. A date for the completion of the literature work/introduction to the project can be agreed early on. There may be other times when project work seems slow e.g. arranging interviews or waiting for responses to questionnaires. Students should be advised to use this time wisely: finalising the introduction to their reports, writing up methods sections, or preparing reference lists. Once the project work starts, they may be very busy. Having sections of the write-up completed will reduce the stress of meeting final deadlines.

Time will be required at the end for writing up. Data collection should end in good time so that the student has time to analyse data, reflect on findings with their supervisor and prepare a quality project report. A date for submission of a full draft of the completed project to the supervisor should be agreed. This should be timed so that it allows the supervisor time to read and comment and make suggestions, as well as for the student to make revisions and prepare their final version. Suggested schedules and goals for meetings are outlined in the next section.

Meetings between supervisors and students

The number of meetings required between supervisors and students will vary greatly from project to project. This will depend on the nature and complexity of the project, and the experience, expertise and confidence of the student. The need for formal meetings will also be influenced by the opportunity for informal contact, which provides a chance to check on progress or respond to minor queries. Thus, the suggestions below are only intended as a guide.

The meetings at the start of any project are important. Time invested at the early stages in setting up the project will usually promote efficient use of time and the achievement of project goals. Time can also pass quickly, so it is helpful at the start to have an overview of the entire project in the overall timescale.

Meeting 1

The initial meeting will be for the student and supervisor to meet each other to share their experiences and goals in terms of the project. At the first meeting the student should be introduced to the subject of the project, which may be new to them, and its broad goals. The supervisor may be able to provide some initial reading, but at the end of the meeting the student should be in a position to embark on their background reading and literature work. Whether or not a systematic literature review is required, the student should have an appreciation of previous research, relevant practice or policy issues to make a case for undertaking the project.

The student may also at this meeting be introduced to the methodological approaches that will be employed in the work. Prior to commencing any fieldwork, they should have an understanding of the methods they will be using and potential problems that might arise. Identifying previous research that has employed similar methods may be helpful in this, as well as referring to texts.

At the end of the meeting there should be a mutual understanding and agreement on what will be achieved prior to the next meeting and a date for this should be arranged. It may also be helpful, at this meeting or the next, to set dates for subsequent meetings. For example, dates could also be agreed for the submission of written work, especially the background and literature work. It is always advisable to aim for early completion of this. A date could be set for the write-up of the study methods. This will help ensure that the writing of the project report is not left to the last minute and enable the student to focus on the results and discussion in the later stages of the work. Supervisors may also find it more convenient not to have all sections of the project submitted for comments at the same time.

The university will usually set a date by which the student must submit their project. The supervisor needs to decide how much time they will need to read and comment on a complete draft, bearing in mind that the student will then need to make revisions before preparing a final version. It may be helpful at the start to suggest a date for submission of the final draft.

When students are new to the setting in which they are undertaking their work, guidance on conduct may be very helpful, as it would be for any visitor. For example, to ensure that they are aware of any dress codes, issues of privacy, departmental routines, priorities of staff, hygiene policies in clinical areas, etc. Orientation to ensure they are familiar with the setting and context can be very helpful.

Meeting 2

At the second meeting progress with background reading and identifying relevant literature can be reviewed. This may lead to the refinement of the aims and objectives and a discussion of the research methods to be employed. Other items to be considered may be meetings with collaborators or progress with applications for permission to conduct the study. A date, and goals, for the next meeting should be agreed.

At this stage, or for the next meeting, depending on the project, supervisors might expect some of the following:

- A plan/draft for the literature review or introduction to the project
- A discussion on methodology and methods that will be employed in the project. This may include possible alternatives, likely pitfalls, potential problems in feasibility, timing or acceptability of data collection, concerns regarding the reliability, validity, completeness of data
- Preparation of a protocol for the study. Depending on the nature of the project, this may cover details on sources of data, methods of data collection and instruments and a plan for analysis
- Development of a Gantt chart identifying activities and milestones with an estimates of their timing

Meeting 3

A further meeting may be required to finalise the methods and operational aspects of the work, and/or to ensure that arrangements are in place for the commencement of project work.

Meeting 4 (+ further meetings as needed)

Subsequent meetings can be arranged as required to check that satisfactory progress is being made. The need for these may depend on the complexity and processes of the study, and whether there are opportunities for informal or chance meetings during the course of the work. Students are likely to be new to many aspects of undertaking research or audit projects. Some (often brief) meetings to ensure that the work is progressing effectively and sensitively may be helpful. During the course of the data collection it will be important to check that the quantity and quality of the data will be adequate to achieve the study objectives.

Meeting 5
Once data collection is complete, meeting to review the data and discuss the plan and procedures for analysis may be helpful.

Meeting 6
Presentation and interpretation of the results is a highlight in many projects. A final meeting may focus on the findings, any further analyses, and the implications. The structure and content of results and discussion sections of the project report can be discussed, along with any other plans for dissemination. Submission of a full draft of the project report and feedback on the draft report with suggestions for revisions would be expected to follow this meeting. A final meeting could be arranged at this point before the submission of the final report.

Following submission, the university would be expected to liaise with supervisors regarding marking the report and their involvement in assessment processes. There will usually be a proforma and clear marking guidelines. The supervisors' role and the timeline for this should be clear. Marking of projects (and usually second marking) often has to be completed fairly soon after submission.

Students may also be required to present the findings of their research at the university, either orally or as a poster. If so, supervisors may wish to discuss the structure, organisation or content of the slides, poster, and/or oral presentation. They may also wish to arrange for the student to present their findings at the practice-based setting.

Writing up: drafts and final report - what should they look like?
Work presented to supervisors for comment should be in a presentable form. Students should take responsibility for the clarity and accuracy of their writing. It can be difficult to review work and comment on the content, argument and critique when trying to make sense of the writing, or when distracted by errors in language. Organisation of material should be logical and easy for the reader to follow. Students should ensure sentence structure, grammar and spellings are correct. Supervisors should not be proofreading.

It is also important, for students and supervisors, that work is submitted on the agreed dates. If students have concerns regarding the standard or style of write-up that is required, they could be encouraged to present a short section for comment and feedback in the interim.

The introduction should be logically organised, using section and subheadings when appropriate. It may include syntheses of empirical research, conceptual or theoretical perspectives, relevant policy or practice issues. It should identify any gaps in knowledge so that it is clear why the project is to be undertaken. The methods section should include a methodology (justification of, and reasons for, the choice of methods with a discussion of their strengths and weaknesses) and a description of the methods, i.e. the procedures employed in their study.

The presentation of the results will depend on the nature of the study and the methods employed. The results may be organised according to the study objectives. The organisation should be logical and the findings clear. The use of tables and charts, or quotes in the case of qualitative studies, is often helpful. These should be accompanied by some textual explanation highlighting key messages. To avoid repetition of the results, the discussion should focus on the implications of the findings. There may be important messages relevant to policy and practice. Relating the findings to the existing literature, perhaps key papers that were identified in the introduction, will indicate how the findings concur with, add to, or contradict our current understanding. An attempt could be made to consider possible reasons for similarities and differences between the study findings and previous studies. There should also be some acknowledgement and discussion of the limitations of the study and possibly some suggestions for future work. The write-up should be comprehensively referenced in a consistent style e.g. Harvard or Vancouver conventions. Making sure that reference lists are complete and in the correct format should be the responsibility of the student.

Overall, students should demonstrate understanding and an ability to critically appraise the literature by highlighting gaps in previous research and presenting a clear argument for why the current study was conducted. They should show an understanding of the methodological approach employed and its scientific basis; whether or not, in the course of the project, they selected and devised the procedures used. They should be able to reflect upon findings of their study in the light of the methodology and consider their value and implications. It should also be the student's responsibility to ensure that they are familiar with the requirements for the presentation of their project report including paper or electronic versions, contents, layout, format, word limits and other specifications.

There is more detailed guidance for students regarding writing-up the project in other chapters.

Conclusion

Undertaking project work in a practice or clinical setting is an immensely valuable experience for students. It allows them to participate in a study that is of relevance to present day patient care. They develop an awareness of the role of research in informing professional practice and medicines use, and they gain an understanding of research methodology in terms of its science and its execution in a real life setting. Without collaboration between tutors in different sectors of pharmacy services and the universities, these valuable educational opportunities could not be offered to our future practitioners.

Questions

1. **What are the advantages of practice-based pharmacy projects for both students and practitioners?**

2. **Which of the following roles would the practice-based supervisor generally be expected to take the lead in? (Select all that apply)**
   A: Identifying projects
   B: Assisting the student in developing a systematic search strategy for their literature review
   C: Assisting the student in gaining local approvals
   D: Overseeing the day-to-day running of the project
   E: Providing training and advice on methods of analysis
   F: Proofreading the draft report

3. **Identify three strategies for ensuring good collaboration between practice-based and university supervisors.**

4. **Which factors should be taken into account when helping students plan their time effectively?**

5. **Identify a strategy that could be used to help students with time planning.**

CHAPTER 7

A scientific approach to your research

LEARNING OBJECTIVES

Upon completion of this chapter you should be able to:

- apply a scientific approach to your pharmacy practice project
- distinguish between methods and methodology
- define the terms reflexivity, reliability, validity and generalisability.

An appreciation of principles of scientific enquiry and research methodology relevant to your discipline is expected for the award of a qualification when studying at masters or post-graduate level. This includes possessing a conceptual understanding that enables you to critically evaluate current research and advanced scholarship, and evaluate and critique relevant methodologies. It is also expected that you can apply this knowledge to select and apply techniques applicable to your own research. You should also be able to demonstrate an understanding of how established techniques of research and enquiry contribute to the development of a discipline its application.

Many smaller projects (especially those undertaken in part fulfilment of requirements for an undergraduate or masters degree) form part of a larger project or research programme. In these cases, many decisions may have already been made regarding the aims, design and methodology of the research. The project may already be underway. However, if this is the case, you should still be able to reflect on principles and practices of scientific enquiry and research methodology in relation to your study. When you come to write-up your project you should be prepared to discuss these issues as they apply to your work.

A feature of research into healthcare, pharmacy practice and medicines use is that it has attracted researchers from a wide range of disciplines. These include pharmacy, sociology, anthropology, psychology, medicine, education, history, epidemiology, demography, policy analysis and economics, among others. Researchers from these disciplines have applied their own scholarship, perspectives and techniques helping to create the broad and stimulating discipline of pharmacy practice research. Approaches and methods from all these disciplines are now applied by pharmacy practice researchers who frequently collaborate with academics and practitioners with a wide range of backgrounds and interests. However, the ultimate goal of pharmacy practice research is to improve our understanding of professional practice and medicines use to inform the development of pharmacy services to meet health and pharmaceutical care needs of patients and the public. Applied research, by its very nature, is often designed to achieve pragmatic rather than theoretical goals. Nevertheless, it is important to demonstrate how the work is underpinned by a scientific approach, which may, or may not, be germane to a particular discipline, and that the findings of the research are clear and dependable.

What is a scientific approach?

The question of the nature and principles of scientific enquiry is a huge subject area in itself, and one which has been addressed and contested from many standpoints. Thus, the goal here is to provide some insights into the way that researchers from different disciplines and perspectives may conceptualise, formulate and address research questions. This may enable you to step back and consider the underlying assumptions and perspectives that surround your own research questions.

Researchers from different disciplines have their own ways of viewing 'their world'. This is sometimes referred to as *ontology* (which has been defined as the study of being or existence). This world view will influence the different approaches that a researcher would take to further their understanding. This is sometimes referred to as *epistemology* (theory of human knowledge). These differing perspectives will in turn influence the questions that they would pose and the methods that they would use in their research.

For example, faced with an issue of mental health in a population, historians, anthropologists, epidemiologists, clinicians and pharmacists bring their own viewpoints regarding the nature of mental health and illness. These perspectives would lead them to develop distinct research agendas to further their knowledge and understanding. Particular types and sources of data may be required. Thus, researchers from the different disciplines would then have their own methodological approaches, or research tools, that they would employ to answer these questions. Different ways of viewing phenomena are often complementary. Thus, in addressing many issues in pharmacy practice and health services research a range of researchers from different disciplines and backgrounds may be involved.

Table 7.1 illustrates some of the differing viewpoints that may be adopted by researchers from different disciplines, together with examples of the sorts of research question that they may formulate and the methods that they may use.

In our learning we are embedded in the perspectives, approaches and methods that distinguish our discipline from others. In our research we often do not acknowledge the role of these perspectives as determinants in the research process. More often we take for granted our ontology and epistemology, and do not stop to reflect on wider or alternative perspectives and approaches. As a consequence, any scientific appraisal tends to focus exclusively on methodology and methods. For your own research, you may like to broaden this to reflect upon:

- your 'world-view' and underlying perspectives and assumptions regarding the nature of your research topic and the type of knowledge that will further your understanding
- how these have led to the formulation of your research question (identification of research priorities)
- what has informed your choice of methods for your study (methodology).

Pharmacy practice and related research is most commonly executed as an applied discipline. However, it may be necessary to view any piece of research in the context of its discipline to appraise its scientific rigour: the

Table 7.1: *Disciplinary approaches to research: an example in mental health*

Discipline	Viewpoint	Research questions	Methods
Anthropologist	Mental health/illness as part of life, viewed and managed in the context of beliefs and norms of a community	To identify relevant health beliefs from the perspective of the community; how mental health/illness is defined explained and/or managed in their natural contexts	Detailed observation and examination by a researcher who lives as a member of the community
Sociologist	Mental health/illness as a part or consequence of wider structures, operation of society and interaction of individuals within	How and why particular population groups may experience better or poorer mental health; factors in society that influence people's experiences of mental health and its management	Social surveys among populations and/or interviews with individuals, to gather information on experiences and views and possible associated factors
Psychologist	Mental health/illness as experienced by the individual	Impact on emotional well-being/self-concept. Decision-making about when to use medicines	Interviews and/or application of structured instruments to gain insights into the beliefs and perspectives of individuals
Epidemiologist/ pharmacoepidemiologist	Patterns of mental health/illness in populations as defined by established measures (often clinical) in populations	The prevalence of mental health problems within a society, comparing different population groups, and identifying associated factors	Analysis of databases that include diagnostic information: patient notes, prescriptions dispensed
Economist	Cost and benefits to society and individuals as a consequence of health status; costs are central to decisions about the provision of healthcare	Costs to individuals, health services and/or society of mental illness and its management	Cost analysis from the perspective of stakeholders; cost-effectiveness/ benefits of mental health programmes
Pharmacologist	Mental health/illness as altered physiological process	Development, and mechanisms of action, of chemotherapeutic agents on relevant cellular processes or neuronal and biochemical pathways	Examination of therapeutic and unwanted effects
Pharmacist	Mental health/illness viewed as altered physiological process modifiable by chemotherapeutic intervention	Use of pharmacotherapy in the management of mental health problems for individual patients	Which patients benefit from medication? Appropriateness/choice of therapy for a patient; monitoring of outcomes

conceptualisation of the research question, the methodological approach and the execution of the work itself.

Reflexivity

Pharmacy practice research and related research is eclectic. Researchers adopt and adapt methods from many disciplines that they deem will be the best way of answering a research question. However, they should not be oblivious of the underlying personal values or viewpoints that they bring. It is important to recognise that others may view any issue in a very different way and prioritise a different set of research questions. Thus, whilst researchers may view themselves as objective investigators, they are in fact an important influence in the research process. This is often more apparent in qualitative research, where the researcher has a major role in directing and redirecting the research throughout the data collection and analysis (see **Chapter 12** and **Chapter 15**). However, a critical appraisal of the values and decisions of the researcher in conceptualising the research question, designing and executing the study, and interpreting the findings is referred to as reflexivity. Engaging in these reflexive activities requires scholarly thought and demonstrates an awareness of some of the difficulties of defining 'objectivity' or claiming a 'scientific' approach to research and the 'knowledge' generated.

In your study you may feel that it would be beneficial to reflect upon:

- your underlying viewpoints and preconceptions that you brought to the research, especially those that will have influenced your aims and objectives (as discussed above)
- the methods you selected and decisions you made to do things in particular ways (throughout the research)
- the effect that these might have had on your findings.

Methodology and methods

Methodology refers to the science or study of methods. Methodology is about the choice and selection of particular methods to answer a research question. The scientific basis and rationale for selecting particular methods (methodology) for any study should be discussed. This may explain, with reasons, your approach (e.g. quantitative or qualitative, study design), choice of methods (existing databases, interviews, observation etc.) and details of study execution and procedures (e.g. populations and samples, instruments, data processing decisions). This discussion of methodology can be distinguished from your *methods*, which is a description of what you actually did.

In your methodology you need to justify your approach and methods in terms of their scientific basis. Say why you have selected them, highlight their strengths and weaknesses, perhaps comparing with alternatives.

All methods have their advantages and disadvantages. You should show an awareness of potential difficulties and problems (e.g. regarding their validity or reliability) and any steps you could take to address them. You have to argue that you have identified the most appropriate methods for achieving your objectives and show that you appreciate any compromises that stem from these choices. For example, you may have to weigh up the value of a detailed study focusing on a small locality with a less comprehensive survey covering a larger geographical area.

Quantitative and qualitative research

In terms of research methodology, probably the most important distinction is that of *quantitative* and *qualitative* methods. Quantitative methods have a much longer history in research into aspects of healthcare and the use of medicines. Nevertheless, qualitative methods are now well established as well as being seen as essential for many research questions.

Researchers who come from health professions, including pharmacists, are generally more familiar with quantitative approaches to enquiry than qualitative approaches. Quantitative studies are those in which the researcher is aiming to quantify phenomena. They may be small or large; local, national or international. In terms of design, studies may be descriptive or experimental.

Examples of quantitative studies may be:

- Assessments of the *frequencies* of events
- Establishing the *proportion* of people in a population/sample who hold particular views or attitudes
- *Audits* of professional practice and use of medicines, requiring assessment against set criteria
- Assessment of *rates* of adherence among particular populations
- The *timing, duration, resources* associated with activities
- A *comparison* of prescribing patterns and rates between hospitals
- Examination of *associations between variables* in a data set, e.g. number of medicines prescribed and reports of medication-related problems, or attitudes and population characteristics or experiences
- Randomised controlled trials in which differences in outcomes between groups are *measured and compared*
- Studies which involve the application of *statistical procedures*

Qualitative studies are considered appropriate for 'how?' and 'why?' questions. They may be used to explore processes and patterns in people's thoughts and behaviour, and/or to examine the operation of services in the context of their particular settings or circumstances. For example, qualitative researchers may investigate how people see or interpret events, or how they make sense of their experiences or the world around them. They may also aim to identify the meanings that people attach to particular situations or explain their priorities and concerns. In these studies, you are exploring the viewpoints of individuals in detail, usually with a small number carefully selected for the sample. You are not trying to establish the numbers of people who think in a particular way or hold certain views, but may be trying to find out *why* they hold these views and how this affects their behaviour.

For example, you may employ a qualitative approach to explore involvement in professional activities from pharmacists' perspectives. This may examine how pharmacists make decisions about whether or not to engage in the activity, to identify beliefs, experiences or attitudes that influence their decisions, and/or to gain insights into constraining or facilitating factors in their practice setting that are important determinants. Detailed qualitative work will not provide an overview of the extent of involvement, but may provide clues regarding possible reasons, problems and barriers from the point of view of practitioners. The findings may inform further research, perhaps with a larger sample to find out (or quantify) the extent to which these perspectives and problems are also experienced by other practitioners.

Thus you can see how qualitative research, which is often exploratory, tries to explain people's thoughts or actions or other events in terms of their belief systems, experiences, situation or circumstances and suggest why different situations may arise. Researchers are aiming to present the viewpoints of respondents as accurately and comprehensively as possible, leaving their own views and preconceptions behind. To achieve this, methods which provide opportunities for respondents to present and explain their individual thoughts, beliefs and behaviours are required. In contrast, in quantitative research the goal is to count events or behaviours, test a hypothesis, and/or quantify relationships between variables or population groups. Predetermined structured instruments are commonly applied.

To gain an understanding of how and why people think and behave in particular ways, qualitative research is often undertaken in the *natural setting*. For example, if you were interested in the sorts of problems people had when using their medicines at home, it might be helpful to visit them at home to collect the data. You could then examine in detail how they use their medicines in the context of their environment and home life, the types of problems they experience, how and why these arise and how they are managed.

Whilst health services research draws on quantitative and qualitative methods, often as part of the same research programme or project, combining these has not been without its controversies. Some researchers believe that combining quantitative and qualitative approaches (or methods or data) ignores the differing epistemological approaches which underpin the research. The distinction between quantitative and qualitative research is sometimes seen as reflecting. On the one hand, a *positivist* world view based on a belief that there is a true state of affairs which can be objectively measured, and on the other, a context-specific social reality in which the qualitative researcher themselves is an actor. Purists may see quantitative and/or qualitative research as representing different *paradigms*: distinct ways of viewing the world with consequences for conceptualisation of problems, and methodologies for the gathering and interpretation of data.

Methodological approaches in quantitative and qualitative research

Many different approaches and methodologies are associated with both quantitative and qualitative research. It is not possible to provide comprehensive coverage here. However, to illustrate the diversity of approaches and methods that have been applied in pharmacy practice and medicines research, a few of the most common are outlined. There are many texts that you can turn to if you wish to explore either the broad subject area or particular approaches in more detail.

Survey research has a wide application across many subject areas and is possibly the most common method in pharmacy practice research. Survey research is viewed as a quantitative approach in which data are collected from a sample of sufficient size and representativeness to enable generalisations to be made to a wider population. Data are usually collected using structured instruments that will have been selected and devised in line with the study objectives. Analysis will usually involve the application of appropriate statistical procedures. Survey data can also be collected in interviews with participants and/or by observation of activities or events in different practice settings. Other sources of survey data may be diverse, e.g. patients' notes, prescriptions dispensed, queries to a helpline, etc. A *census* differs from a survey in that data are collected from the entire population rather than a sample.

Epidemiological research often relies on data in existing databases. It is a population-based approach in which statistical procedures are employed to examine patterns of disease, health needs, service uptake, prescribing, etc. according to predetermined objectives. *Pharmacoepidemiology* employs similar methods but with a more specific focus on issues related to the use of medicines.

Experimental studies, in particular randomised controlled trials (RCTs), are central to the development of an evidence base to guide the provision and delivery of healthcare and the use of medicines. These employ experimental design (see **Chapter 9**) which is characterised by carefully controlled conditions and are designed to ensure that all variables except those under study are equivalent in the experimental and control groups. These studies also apply tight eligibility criteria in the selection of participants. RCTs conducted and reported according to established guidelines, e.g. those of the CONSORT group (*www.consort-statement. org*), are often seen as a gold standard in 'objective' research, generating dependable data distinguishing different treatment regimens as measured by specific outcomes. However, the place of RCTs as a 'gold standard' is contested. The strictly controlled eligibility criteria often narrow outcome measures and are believed to represent an artificial setting; that is one that does not necessarily take into account the different patient groups and environments in which any treatment or intervention may be applied. Thus, a study provides objective evidence in relation to a specific hypothesis (the effectiveness of an intervention when compared with a control or other course of action) which it was designed to test. However, the study findings may not be applicable to other patient groups, settings, circumstances, etc. that were outside the study criteria. Experimental studies are sometimes seen as *reductionist* in that they are focused on a particular predetermined outcome measure. Some researchers see this as a limitation of randomised controlled trials, arguing that a more *holistic* approach to the evaluation of an intervention has advantages. An example of this is *realistic evaluation*. A more holistic approach may include the gathering of contextual data relating to the operation and wider outcomes of an intervention, contextual factors that are pertinent to the outcomes in different settings, and circumstances (which may have to be controlled or excluded in an RCT to enable valid statistical comparisons). There may also be factors that are important to the feasibility or success of a particular intervention that will not necessarily be identified by a tightly structured RCT.

A *reductionist* approach breaks down and examines a process or situation in terms of its different components, and studies each one independently of the others or the wider context. In contrast, a *holistic* approach assumes that 'the whole is greater than the sum of the parts' and endeavours to examine a process or event from different perspectives within the same project. Research in which a holistic approach is taken can be complex. To enable an examination from a range of perspectives a number of different approaches and/or methods may be required. This is referred to as triangulation (see **Chapter 9**). Not uncommonly, both qualitative and quantitative methods may be employed.

A feature of holistic research is that it is generally concerned with an examination of behaviours or events, taking contextual factors into account. *Ethnography* refers to the study of individuals in their natural setting to characterise and provide potential explanations for particular events and behaviours. It is a qualitative methodology that aims to provide systematic and detailed evidence to explain phenomena in the light of structural and organisational factors, actions and interactions, personal experiences and views. A mixture of methods may be applied in an ethnographic study.

Phenomenology is a qualitative approach that focuses on meanings. It is concerned with individuals and how they see or interpret situations and events in the world around them. A phenomenological approach aims to examine events and actions from the perspective of the individuals under study, understand their interpretations of events and situations and how these lead to different beliefs, actions and behaviours. Thus, phenomenology is concerned with *interpretation* and individuals' *constructions* of reality. This can be contrasted with *positivism* in that instead of trying to explain events and situations in an 'objective' way, it assumes that behaviours and events are a consequence of an individual's beliefs, 'ways of seeing', meanings they attach to phenomena, and ultimately their constructions of their own realities.

Thus *positivism* (a belief in a 'true' state of affairs that can be objectively (scientifically) measured) and *constructionism* (including phenomenology) are illustrative of the diverse approaches of quantitative and qualitative research paradigms that are applied in research into health and medicines. It should also be recognised that different terms, their meanings and definitions have also been, and remain, the subject of debate. Furthermore, philosophy and methodology are evolving and not static fields. The philosophy of science, nature of scientific enquiry and what constitutes scientific knowledge is a huge subject matter beyond the scope of this text, and one which has engaged philosophers and scientists, and presented many schools of thought over the centuries. You may wish to delve further.

Principles of validity and reliability

Whatever the methodological approach, questions of scientific rigour arise. The concepts of reliability and validity are pertinent to all studies. An understanding of these concepts enables you to achieve and demonstrate a scientific approach.

Potential threats to the reliability and validity of research arise in relation to all stages of the research process: sampling procedures, data collection, instruments and measures, data processing and analysis, and all types of study. They are discussed in different chapters at the appropriate points. Throughout your project work you should apply critical thought to your methods and findings to ensure that you are realistic about the quality and integrity of the data. You need to feel confident of your interpretation of the findings and that you are not overstating any conclusions or the potential value of the work.

Reliability

Reliability refers to the extent to which procedures, measures and data are reproducible or internally consistent.

Problems of reliability may arise in relation to repeated measures on a piece of diagnostic equipment, uniformity between researchers in the collection of data, adherence of interviewers to an interview schedule, completeness in maintaining records of non-responders, care and attentiveness when observing events, consistency to questions in a questionnaire, agreement between researchers in the coding of data, etc. Problems of reliability can emerge at all stages in research. In the development of research instruments, data collection procedures, and data processing and analysis, potential problems with regard to the reliability of data must be identified and addressed. Poor reliability at any stage can undermine the value of the work and dependability of the study findings. It is important to keep an open mind and be alert to any concerns. Problems can often not be ironed out completely, but it is important that you, as the researcher, identify difficulties. You are then in a position to take steps to address problems and/or assess their implications for the findings of the study.

Validity

Validity refers to the extent to which the findings of a study are a true reflection of phenomena under study. Do the instruments (e.g. questions in an interview, records maintained by an observer) actually measure what they are designed to measure?

All methods and studies present their own concerns with regard to validity. As with reliability, potential questions regarding validity can arise at all stages of the research process. It is essential for the ultimate value of the research that they are identified and addressed. Threats to validity that arise with different methods and at different stages of a project will be highlighted in later chapters.

Potential problems in validity arise in particular in relation to data collection and the development of instruments. In observation studies, it is recognised that people when being observed may purposely or inadvertently change their behaviour; data will not then be an accurate reflection of the true situation. In an interview, respondents may be reluctant to discuss certain relevant issues or present a negative viewpoint, thus leading to biased information. In self-completion questionnaires, respondents may tend to underestimate on some variables (e.g. their smoking habits) and overestimate on others.

Most studies require measurement of phenomena. Demonstrating that any measure is a valid reflection of a variable on interest can be difficult. Physiological measures are used in clinical medicine, but may or may not provide a reliable or valid indication of the severity of a condition or its impact.

Finding valid measures of some variables is not straightforward. Variables that are difficult to define will inevitably present problems for researchers. For example, health inequalities are high on many governments' agendas. Thus, health services researchers will usually want to gather data that enable an examination of experiences of individuals of different socio-economic status. To examine any associations between socio-economic status and health, or the use of medicines, requires its measurement. Although socio-economic status is a concept that is widely recognised, it is a complex construct and is difficult to define. Various approaches have been used as 'proxy' measures in survey research to measure socio-economic status. These include questions about occupation, education, income, other lifestyle factors, and/or combinations of these. However, questions remain regarding the extent to which these measures are accurate (valid) reflections of what is generally recognised as socio-economic status. Similar problems arise in the classification of people according to ethnicity; how can people be grouped in a way that is a valid reflection of their cultural identity?

Health status and health-related quality of life are important measures in much research. Measurement is complex. Individuals differ in their perceptions of their own health. In assessment of health-related quality of life, peoples lives are compromised in different ways as a consequence of their health status and each person may differ in the aspects of their health that are most important to them. Conceptual, theoretical and practical problems in the measurement of these variables have attracted many researchers. As a consequence, there are many validated measures that can be employed.

Variables relating to the use of medicines can also be complex. For example, a number of methods have been used to measure compliance with, or adherence to, medicines regimens. Firstly, a conceptual issue may arise which may influence the approach of the researcher. An assessment of 'compliance' might be a measure of the extent to which an individual follows instructions. The concept of adherence recognises that the perspectives of individuals will influence on their use of medicines. Thus, in studies of 'adherence' researchers often focus on patients' perspectives and measures reflect their role in decision-making regarding the use of their medicines. Accordingly, there are a range of measures of compliance/ adherence that are commonly employed, all with their own strengths and limitations. These include records of refills from pharmacies, counting of doses remaining in a container, electronic devices to detect use of a product, physiological measures and self-reports. Other concepts or constructs employed by researchers into pharmacy and medicines that present difficulties include measures of potential severity of medicine-related problems, the quality of advice, self-efficacy in the management of illness and use of medicines.

In recent decades, measurement of complex variables in health services research has been an important focus of many methodologists. As a result, there are now many measures in the literature which have been developed and validated using rigorous approaches. In general, if you wish to measure a complex variable, it is better to look for, and adopt, an existing measure than attempt to devise your own.

Generalisability (external validity)

The generalisability (sometimes referred to as the external validity) is concerned with the extent to which the findings of a study can be applied to individuals beyond the sample. Many studies involve samples rather than a whole population. Studies are often focused on a single location or a small number of areas, but there may be a strong argument that the findings have wider relevance.

The most important issues that determine the generalisability of study findings are the sampling strategies, procedures, sizes and response rates (e.g. surveys), representativeness, and completeness of data (e.g. databases). Assuming probability sampling procedures, comprehensiveness of databases and sampling frames, good response rates, and validity of data, then findings should be generalisable to the population from which the sample was drawn. In addition to this, for many studies researchers may wish to address the issue of generalisability to populations beyond the sampling frame. There may be strong arguments for claiming that much wider generalisation is valid.

Conclusion

Your research project can provide an opportunity for you to engage in scholarship at the forefront of your discipline and/or participate in the creation of new knowledge that will be relevant to professional practice and patient care. This work will require an appreciation of conceptual, theoretical and practical perspectives regarding the generation and interpretation of data within a discipline. Reflection on the scientific basis of your research questions methodology and methods will enhance your understanding of the research process.

Questions

1. Why is important to take a scientific approach to your project?

2. Explain the difference between methods and methodology.

3. Consider the experiences and perspectives that you bring to your pharmacy practice project and how these may impact on the findings.

4. Which one of the following may cause a reduction in the reliability of a study?
   A: Different students who are carrying out observations interpreting items on a data collection instrument differently
   B: Participants completing a questionnaire interpreting a question differently to how the researchers intended them to

5. What is generalisability?

CHAPTER 8

Reviewing the literature

LEARNING OBJECTIVES

Upon completion of this chapter you should be able to:

- identify different types of literature review
- develop a search strategy
- understand the principles of critical appraisal of studies.

While different types of literature reviews will be appropriate for different studies, taking a step-by-step approach to identifying and reviewing relevant literature is a key early component of any study. This aids in the development of the aims and objectives of the study and in devising a suitable methodology for meeting the objectives. As discussed in **Chapter 3**, a well conducted literature review (*Box 8.1*) will provide you with a good overview of the extent of research on a particular subject, the range of topics that have been examined, and the level of current knowledge. It will help you to define your own research objectives that build on existing knowledge and/or fill in any important gaps. You will also find out about the different methods that previous researchers have used to study your topic. If they have highlighted the strengths and weaknesses of their methods, this may be helpful to you in planning your own study.

Box 8.1: A comprehensive literature review

- It is important to ensure that the work builds on existing theories or knowledge, and that it does not duplicate the work of others. It will help ensure that your work extends our knowledge or understanding in specific ways.
- It allows the identification of factors that have been found by other researchers to be important to the topic or issues under study, so they can be taken into account. These may relate to the setting of the research, particular structural or organisational factors or factors relevant to particular population groups.
- It enables the identification of the perspectives of different stakeholders, so that they can be considered.
- It assists in selecting the best methods for the study. There may be a number of ways of obtaining data relevant to the study objectives, all of which will have their strengths and weaknesses. Review of the methods used by others enables you to identify different options, together with their advantages and disadvantages, when planning your own study.

Different types of literature reviews can be conducted depending on the purpose of the review. A systematic review will aim to systematically identify and critically review all literature that meets a set of predefined inclusion criteria. In contrast, a scoping review will set out to review a broader range of literature in less depth. For example, its purpose may be to identify areas that have been researched in relation to a study area and where there may begaps. It will provide a general overall picture, rather than an in-depth focus on a more specific area. Sometimes a scoping review may be carried out before a systematic review in order to identify areas that a systematic review should focus on.

The stages of conducting a literature review are discussed under three main headings: finding relevant material, organisation of documents and critical appraisal. The processes of these are also summarised in *Box 8.2*.

Box 8.2: The stages of a literature review

Finding relevant material
- Describe your search strategy – approach and general plan for finding relevant material including the types of material/evidence for which you will be looking.
- Describe the details of your search procedures (implementation of your strategy), e.g. which databases, keywords, journals, searches of citations; what was successful and what was not; what you found and how/if this informed further stages of your search. How successful do you think you were in identifying all important and relevant material?

Organisation and review
- Organise the papers/documents that you find into topic areas, so that you can describe, review, synthesise and summarise the findings across studies for each topic. You will then be in a position to present an overview of current knowledge in each. You should aim to bring together the findings of different studies yourself; don't just provide a separate summary of each paper and expect the reader to synthesise into a body of evidence.
- Demonstrate an appreciation of different types of evidence and their value in informing current knowledge regarding any topic area, e.g. commentaries, reports, peer-reviewed research all have their own place and value.

Critical appraisal
- Demonstrate an ability to 'critically appraise' research. All research presents difficulties and compromises in its execution. Acknowledge the strengths and weaknesses of previous work and take this into account when reporting the findings of studies. Distinguish good and more important studies from those that are less valuable.
- Provide an overview of the extent of our knowledge in relation to your topic, in terms of both the range of issues that have been researched and the quality of the evidence. Indicate important gaps and possible questions for future work (which may include your own!).

Finding relevant material

Finding material is fundamental for the success of any literature review. You want to avoid a situation in which relevant work is missed that would have been valuable in informing your study objectives. In pharmacy practice research this can be problem because of the interdisciplinary nature of many studies. Frequently, issues relevant to the study objectives may relate to professional practice, clinical issues and problems, and/ or social science perspectives. These issues may have been addressed by researchers from different health professions, e.g. nursing, medicine and others as well as pharmacy, or from different academic disciplines, e.g. health psychology, epidemiology, sociology, etc. This may affect where the work is published and means that, in conducting the literature review, a wide range of databases, libraries and journals may have to be explored. As a result of the multidisciplinary and collaborative nature of much health service and pharmacy practice research, searching may have to extend to specialist clinical areas, social science databases, etc. Depending on the topic area, it can add to the value of a study if the possibility of contributions from other disciplines is considered. It may be worth keeping an open mind. Theoretical perspectives can provide an additional dimension to a research problem and sometimes a framework for the conceptualisation of a study.

In identifying relevant papers, it can be helpful to think in terms of a two-stage process: a *search strategy* and a *search procedure*. When you come to write up the methods for your literature review, you can explain them separately.

Your search strategy

The search strategy refers to your overall approach to looking for relevant literature. For example, you may decide that you need to search in the literature of a number of different disciplines.

Databases

Due to its wide scope and interdisciplinary nature, a review of the literature into medicines use and pharmacy practice may draw on a variety of databases. Those often used include: PubMed, a publicly available version of MEDLINE which is a source of abstracts of peer-reviewed research into biomedical sciences; articles relating to broad clinical topics, health and healthcare drawn from medical, nursing and allied health disciplines such as EMBASE (Excerpta Medica database) which covers wide-ranging literature in biomedical science and pharmaceutical research and; research into healthcare and the use of medicines across different disciplines such as IPA (International Pharmaceutical Abstracts) which focuses on pharmaceutical sciences, pharmacy practice and medicines use. The

Cochrane database is a library of high-quality, systematic reviews that aim to support evidence-based healthcare. Depending on the topic of your research, you may decide to investigate other sources, e.g. psychology, education or specialist clinical sources. Other databases that may be of interest are the British Nursing Index (BNI) and CINAHL which focus on nursing and allied health professionals, IBSS is a bibliography of the social sciences, ERIC is a source of documents on research and practice in education and PsychINFO covers psychology research and practice including material that of health focus. Various citation indexes which enable the searching of reference lists or 'citations' provide an additional means of identifying relevant material. Sometimes independent, special interest organisations maintain their own libraries or databases of relevant material which can be very helpful in highlighting topical issues and providing insights into new developments in research, practice and policy.

Developing search terms

Identifying the right search terms is key to finding relevant material. This is not always straightforward, especially projects that span subject areas, or where material might have been written and placed to reach a range of diverse audiences. It can sometimes be difficult to ensure that all the best search terms have been identified. However, there are several strategies that can help.

PICO

Firstly, breaking your research question down into separate components. The PICO framework is used to organise a clinical question into components parts, but it can also be used to break down a literature search topic.

P = Population, Patient Group or Problem
I = Intervention
C = Comparator or Control (if appropriate)
O = Outcome

Once you have identified each component, the next stage is to spend some time brainstorming related terms or phrases. During this phase you will need to consider synonyms and related terms (e.g. concordance or adherence), variant spelling (e.g. apnoea or apnea), broader topic areas (e.g. apnoea or apnea or respiratory diseases or respiratory conditions) and pluralisation (e.g. disease or diseases).

These terms and phrases will become your search terms (also known as search commands) when you search a database. All databases and search engines provide wildcards and truncation symbols to help you cluster words, e.g. an * at the end of a word will retrieve all words with variant stem-spelling: disease* = disease or diseases or diseased. The help pages or field guides of the individual databases give specific advice about wildcards.

The best practice searching of databases is to search the components separately generating x number of clusters, then combining the clusters at the end. Using PICO will generate 3-4 clusters. A useful analogy is cake-baking. Throwing all the ingredients of a cake into a mixing bowl at the same time will lead to uncertain results. Instead, preparing the individual ingredients separately will allow greater control and comprehension of the process.

Subject headings

The content of many databases including MEDLINE, EMBASE and CINAHL is indexed with subject headings. Subject headings describe the content of the articles that the database record summarises.

Taking MEDLINE as an example, an indexer will read a candidate article and then map its key topics or features to three or more subject headings, which MEDLINE calls descriptors. These descriptors are derived from a controlled vocabulary called medical subject headings (MeSH) and entered into the subject heading field, which is called MeSH terms. Controlled vocabularies operate like thesauri in which synonymous words are designated to a subject heading. MeSH terms are organised into sixteen hierarchical structures called trees.

For all databases that utilise them, extracting the correct subject heading from the thesaurus and adding it the subject heading field in the database help ensure the search retrieves relevant results. Significantly, consulting a controlled vocabulary can help with the brainstorming of search terms thanks to its tree-like structure. A very broad category, e.g. diseases, serves as a large and rooted trunk from which more slender branches bloom. Each offshoot yields more, the fineness of a branch representing the specificity of a topic. Viewing a tree enables a searcher to broaden, focus or extend a search by exploiting its subject heading context.

Using Cochrane

Many of the systematic reviews published by the Cochrane Library will include the search strategies used by the researchers. The strategies may be narratively described in the introduction or methodology sections of the reviews, or presented in full in appendices. In addition, retrieved results on the list pages feature PICO panels. These can be mined when brainstorming or applicable sections of a strategy can be reused when searching.

Peer-to-peer review

As at any stage of a research project, asking a peer, supervisor or team member to review your selection of search terms is important. They may not be able to ratify your choices but questions they may pose could stimulate further brainstorming or processing.

Developing inclusion and exclusion criteria

You need to decide about different types of material or evidence (*Table 8.1*) that you need for your review. Developing inclusion and exclusion criteria can help you take a systematic approach to selecting relevant material. These criteria will relate to both the studies that you will include and the publication types that you will include.

Criteria related to the studies may include the scope of the topic area, the study design, and the population that will be included, amongst other things. For example, you may decide you will include all study designs or limit your review to a specific type of study design, such as a randomised controlled trial. You may decide to focus on a specific population, such as those with a specific condition or in a specific age range, or you may wish to include a broader population.

In terms of publication type, you will need to make decisions about whether or not to include publications not written in English. In addition, you may decide to restrict your search to published (peer-reviewed) literature, or alternatively believe that you should try to find work that may be of sufficient quality, but not yet published - known as 'grey literature'. It may be appropriate to broaden the scope of the literature work to include material that, if not scientifically rigorous, still provides insights into relevant issues and perspectives for the topic of study. In healthcare research there will often be individuals and groups who have written about the problems that you are researching from their perspectives. Thus, in addition to research studies that are published in academic and professional journals, other types of document may be informative and valuable in planning the study. Therefore, you may wish to include commentaries, e.g. by practitioners, researchers or other interested individuals, discussion articles written to promote debate, letters to journals, policy documents or material produced by various stakeholder groups. Special interest groups (professional and non-professional), government bodies and local health organisations may undertake research and/or produce documents representing their views and priorities. Exploration of a wide range of sources helps to ensure that the groundwork for the study is as comprehensive as possible. See *Table 8.1* for an overview of different types of evidence, their sources and application.

Table 8.1: *Types of evidence*

Evidence	Possible sources	Application
Opinions of individuals	As expressed in correspondence/editorials in professional and/or academic journals	May assist in identifying issues relevant to particular stakeholders
Opinions of experts	As expressed in correspondence/editorials in professional and/or academic journalsl	Identification of accepted viewpoints and/or difficulties and controversies in interpretation of evidence
Journalistic investigation	Newspapers, websites, professional journals	Controversies regarding subject area; on-the-ground experiences of individuals
Scholarly discussion presenting informed arguments and perhaps applying inductive or deductive thought	Peer-reviewed academic journals, reports of specialist organisations/expert bodies	Application of theory and its development in shedding light on phenomena
Small local research studies	Peer-reviewed research in professional or academic journals, studies reported in other journals/publications, reports for local practitioners or stakeholders	Depends on the scientific rigour, but may be of value to local setting and possibly of wider relevance
Larger research studies	Peer-reviewed academic or professional journals	Assuming scientific rigour, evidence should be dependable and applicable to wider populations
Systematic reviews of the literature: following rigorous methodology	Peer-reviewed academic or professional journals Cochrane database	Valuable, providing an overview of the extent and quality of evidence on a given topic, but may be narrow in scope and the range of material included
Meta-analyses: statistical analysis of data that have been combined from a number of previous studies, of sufficient methodological similarity, on a given topic	Peer-reviewed journals	If conducted in scientific manner can provide valuable and generalisable results. The technique can be limited because of heterogeneity between studies and/or insufficient information relating to procedures and measures employed
Policy papers and guidelines; reports of specialist organisations	Professional bodies, government, think-tanks, non-governmental organisations, consumer organisations	Often informative, well researched and/or based on expert opinions. May be designed and written to present a particular viewpoint or argue a case, so need to question partiality. May present insights into topical issues. Generally not subject to peer-review processes
Unpublished projects and research	Those of undergraduate- and postgraduate students, local project work	These documents may provide helpful insights in the topic areas and/or highlight difficulties of research in these areas

Decisions about inclusion and exclusion criteria will be decided based on a number of factors including the aims and objectives of the project, the volume of literature in your study area, and pragmatic considerations. If there is a large amount of previous work in your area, you may decide to carry out a more focused strategy. However, if there is not much relevant specific research, including a broader range of literature could be helpful in providing context for your study. You also need to consider the time available for you to carry out your literature review and the number of papers you will have time to review. This will vary between universities but typically 5-10 key papers should be sufficient for most masters projects. Including papers in languages other than English may also be pragmatic if you know the language yourself, have friends or family who can help you translate, or have the resources to pay for an official translation.

When writing up your project report, you should both describe and justify your search strategy; that is, to be clear about *what* you are looking for and *why*. Once you have developed and justified your search strategy, you then need to plan your procedure for finding relevant material.

Your search procedure

The literature search should be as systematic as possible. Online databases are the principal sources for many reviews; they are a valuable starting point. However, in much health services and pharmacy practice research these have to be combined with other approaches; not all journals in which relevant material may appear are included in databases of published research. In particular, articles in non-academic, professional or special interest journals may be a useful source.

Sometimes, a few key papers might be identified from a database which provide a lead for further searches. Particular research teams or authors with an interest in an area could be a focus for a search. You may find that research on particular topics tends to be concentrated in particular journals. The contents and references cited in these relevant papers may provide useful pointers to further important work. Thus, after a database search you may undertake a systematic search of the contents/abstracts pages of particular journals (which may be available online) to identify other relevant work.

Records of all searches should be kept, whether or not these were productive. This should include the databases you have used, search terms, years of publication, restrictions regarding language, and any other decisions you have made regarding eligibility criteria to enable you to select relevant articles. For example, in a systematic review of research, the selection of papers may be restricted to those that meet specific criteria, e.g. publication in a peer-reviewed journal or criteria relating to the scientific quality of the research.

You should also report on other approaches you have used. These may be use of the internet, use of search engines, visiting of particular libraries, searchers of key journals or other publications, contacting specialist organisations or individual experts, etc.

As you conduct your review you should maintain a careful record of what you find at each stage. You should keep a full record of all references that you may include in your review (*Box 8.3*). It can be frustrating in the final stages of the work, when you are busy completing the work, to discover that some of your references are incomplete or that you cannot remember the source of a particular piece of information. Tracing original articles and sources can be difficult and time-consuming. It is wise to make sure you maintain records of the names and initials of all authors, title of article and publication; if a journal, volume: page numbers and year; for other publications year and place of publication and name of publisher. Online sources should provide the weblink and date accessed. There are free online reference management tools that you could use to help you organise your references such as EndNote Online, Zotero and Mendeley.

Box 8.3: Maintaining records of your sources and references

- Journal articles: names with initials of all authors, year of publication, title of article, full title of journal, volume number, first and last page numbers
- Books: names with initials of all authors, year of publication, title of book, place of publication, publisher
- Book chapters in an edited (as opposed to authored) book: the author(s) of the chapter with their initials, the chapter number, title of the chapter and first and last page numbers; the names with initials of the editor(s), year of publication, the title of the book, place of publication, publisher
- Policy document or document from other public or private body: names with initials of all authors (which may be an organisation or individuals on behalf of an organisation), year of publication, title of document, place of publication, publisher
- Website: name of organisation, date of publication and/or date information accessed, title of article (if applicable), web address
- Personal communications: names/affiliations of individuals, names of organisations as appropriate and dates

Organisation and review

The titles and/or abstracts of many articles will be sufficient to indicate whether or not it is likely to be relevant. For those papers that appear to meet the criteria, the full papers will usually be required. A prisma diagram can be helpful in showing the reader of your review the step-by-step approach you have taken to selecting your papers. This is a flowchart which shows a detailed breakdown of your search, including which databases were searched, how many papers were identified, how many duplicates between databases were removed, how many were excluded at the title and abstract stage and how many were excluded after obtaining the full paper. It will also show the papers obtained though routes other than online databases (*Figure 8.1*).

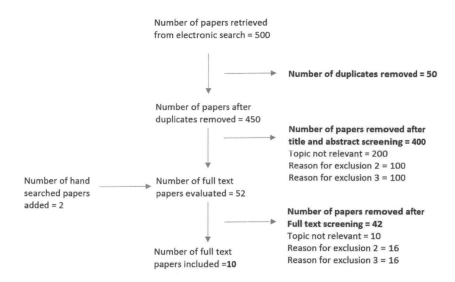

Figure 8.1: *Example of a PRISMA diagram*

Data extraction

Once you have chosen your papers, the next stage is data extraction. You will need to decide what the important information is that you need to extract from each paper. This will vary from study to study and will be partly dependent on your aims and objectives. However, data extraction would typically include study design, study population, country, setting, sample size, outcome measures and key findings. You may find it helpful to tabulate your data extraction processes (*Table 8.2*).

Table 8.2: *Example of a data extraction table template*

Study	Country	Design	Population	Sample size	Outcome measures	Key findings

You need to find a way of presenting the findings of your literature search that enables you to provide an overview of extent of material for each of your research questions or topics of your review. You may start by grouping the papers into different topics or headings; this may be according to the topic area of the article and/or the type of evidence (as in *Table 8.1*). Such an overview can be useful both to you, in organising your material, and also to others as it provides a summary of the extent of relevant published material and the different types of documents. For example, you may have found six research studies of which four were descriptive studies.

In the case of a review of previous research, you will also need to provide a critique of the relevance and quality of the studies (e.g. study setting, design, size and methodology of the study) so that you are able to provide a summary of the evidence derived across all relevant work. It is important to bring the studies together and compare the findings of each. You should consider how and why findings from the studies are similar and different. Based on this appraisal of the literature you should be able to present a summary of the extent of knowledge on your topic, the strengths/weaknesses of the evidence and questions/topics for further investigation.

Critical appraisal

Critical appraisal is an important component of any review of the literature. It is widely acknowledged that research studies (including those in high-quality peer-reviewed journals) vary in their quality and value. It is important to remember that to some extent the findings of all studies are 'an artifact of the methods' employed. An important part of any literature review is to make your own assessment of the strength of the study and the importance of the findings. In making this assessment you might consider the perspectives, contexts and methods of a study. For example, a study may have demonstrated an enhanced pharmacy service improved outcomes for a particular group of patients, but rather than take the conclusions at face value, you may make your own assessment of the scientific approach and the robustness of the methodology. You may ask your own questions about the underlying assumptions of the researchers that may have influenced their research questions and methods. The wider relevance (generalisability) of the findings may be influenced by the population group, study setting, sample size and representativeness. Which patient outcomes were examined? Were the measures appropriate? Are there unanswered questions about feasibility or costs? You could appraise all aspects of the methods and execution of the study and then form a view on the quality of the study and the likely value of the findings.

Thus, when reviewing research papers, the findings and conclusions of a study must be interpreted in the context of the methods used. You should reflect on the study design, sampling procedures, response rates, methods, instruments, measures, analytical processes, issues of reliability and validity, etc. as discussed in other chapters. In terms of methodology, all studies will have their strengths and weaknesses. Compromises are often inevitable and they arise for all sorts of reasons, such as limited time or resources, ethical constraints, low response rates, and/or unforeseen difficulties that arise in the execution of the study. All research presents its own challenges and difficulties. It is important to be able to draw out what is good and valuable in any piece of work and not to focus only on criticism. Thus, by engaging in critical appraisal you are able to take a balanced view regarding the extent to which you think the study is of value and the conclusions are justified, and its place in your review of the literature.

There are a number of tools that have been developed to help you assess the quality of different types of study. These may be helpful in guiding you through the critical appraisal process. For example, the Critical Appraisal Skills Programme (CASP) has developed several tools. CASP tools may not cover all study types used in health services research and pharmacy practice and other tools are also available. It is important to choose a tool which fits the study you are evaluating. When using critical appraisal tools, it may be that not all items are relevant to your study. In general, these tools are best used a guide to the areas of critique that maybe relevant for different types of study.

Alongside an assessment of the quality of the research and the robustness of the methodology, the value of a study in terms of the relevance of its research question or aim needs to be considered. Is the focus of any paper of direct relevance to your own objectives and/or of some indirect relevance?

A step beyond critical appraisal: the literature as a source of data

Literature sources can provide a source of material for further analyses. Data in published studies (and sometimes those which have not yet been published, if they can be located) can be combined to form a new dataset. Bringing together data or results from previous quantitative studies can provide a larger pool of data to which analytical procedures can be applied (*Box 8.4*). This is referred to as *meta-analysis* (see **Chapter 14**). Findings based on a larger dataset can increase the strength (dependability and generalisability) of the findings. Strict criteria regarding quality and focus are applied to the selection of papers. However, in practice the value can be limited because of the inevitable variation in the quality of studies and diversity in methodology.

Techniques for combining the findings of previous qualitative studies can also be applied to qualitative research. These studies may provide a useful resource for further systematic analysis. Sometimes referred to as narrative synthesis, the analysis may be structured to answer a new research question. It will often be informed by a theoretical framework. In addition to the application of data synthesis to qualitative research, similar techniques may also be applied to policy or documents or other documentary sources.

Increasingly, systematic reviews, sometimes including reappraisal or further analyses of data, are providing valuable research evidence. Collection of data is resource-intensive for funders, researchers and participants. Exploiting data to its full potential should be a priority. However, as for any research, it requires the application of rigorous and scientific approaches. Analysis of secondary datasets is discussed further in **Chapter 14**.

Box 8.4: Overview of stages of a literature review and writing up

- Write a general introduction to topic area, leading into a statement of your aims and objectives.
- Provide details of your search strategy and procedure.
- Group the papers that you have found according to your objectives so that you can report on the numbers of papers/articles or other documents that you found that met your search criteria. This will also include information on the types of paper.
- Extract important information from each paper.
- Critically appraise each paper taking into account the type and quality of evidence that it presents, the methodology employed or the sources of information on which it draws. This will enable you to comment on the extent to which you believe the findings and conclusions are supported and justified, and consider the value of the paper to your overall objectives.
- For each group of papers, write a summary that provides an overview of our current knowledge across all relevant studies. This should provide the reader with an overview of the extent of literature on a topic, the type of article or numbers of studies that have been conducted, and the quality of the research. You could highlight any consensus or controversies regarding the subject area or the evidence on any topic and, also, gaps in the literature and priorities for further research.

Conclusion

Conducting a literature review for the first time can be a challenging task, but having a good appreciation of the literature around the subject of your project will help you understand the place of your work and its potential value. Undertaking a literature review also builds other skills. Drawing on a range of different sources to find relevant material you will develop an understanding of the place and value of different types of evidence. You will develop skills in critical appraisal which will require an appreciation of science behind research methodology. Published (and to some extent unpublished) research can be a valuable resource for further interrogation and analysis; again robust scientific approaches must be applied.

Questions

1. What is a scoping review?

2. What is a systematic review?

3. Identify three databases which are commonly searched in pharmacy practice literature reviews.

4. Describe how you might approach developing a search strategy for the literature review for your project.

5. Which one of the following is true?
   A: All items on a critical appraisal tool will be relevant to all studies
   B: Critical appraisal tools will include all relevant aspects of critique for your study
   C: Critical appraisal tools can act as a guide when critically appraising a study

Study design

This chapter provides an overview of the different types of study design features that are commonly employed in pharmacy practice and related research. The 'design' of a study refers to its overall structure as cross-sectional, longitudinal, prospective, retrospective, descriptive, experimental, etc. As discussed in **Chapter 7** there may be many differing approaches and methodologies that could be adopted in research on any topic. Some of these are associated with particular types of study design (*Box 9.1*). However, the principal determinant of the design of any study is the research question or aim.

Box 9.1: Some terms used to define research design and types of study

Audit	Hypothesis generating
Before and after	Hypothesis testing
Case study	Intervention
Cohort	Longitudinal
Cross-sectional	Pilot study
Descriptive	Prevalence
Experimental	Prospective
Exploratory	Quasi-experimental
Feasibility	Randomised controlled trial (RCT)
Holistic	Retrospective

Descriptive studies

The aim of these studies is to document or portray (i.e. describe) phenomena, e.g.:

- Characteristics or practices of a population group
- Activities undertaken by pharmacists or other health professionals
- Behaviour of consumers with regard to their health or medicines
- Views or attitudes of individuals
- Frequencies of events or prevalence of problems

Descriptive studies are important when there is no systematic information (*Box 9.2*). It is true that, for many of the activities that are undertaken in relation to pharmacy services or the use of medicines, we may believe that we have a good idea about what happens. Even if there is no systematic research, we may feel that, based on our own experience, that of our peers' or anecdotal reports, we can estimate the frequency of different types of event in a health or pharmacy setting. We may believe that we have a good idea of the extent of certain health-related behaviours, the range of concerns of individuals with regard to particular issues, or how commonly particular views are held. However, if there is no systematic and accurate documentation of these phenomena, we cannot be sure about the true picture. If the sampling procedures are unscientific or unclear, we cannot (with any certainty) draw inferences and generalise the information to other groups of people or settings. Also, without systematic study we would not have adequate information to investigate any associations between an issue of interest and other factors (e.g. whether or not certain groups of patients are more likely to experience problems with their medicines, or whether there are any associations between the location of pharmacies and the demand for different services) with a known degree of accuracy.

> ## Box 9.2: Descriptive studies
>
> - Provide important data for informing people inside and outside the profession about pharmacy services and the use of medicines, and how and why these may vary
> - Enable the assessment of whether services are meeting healthcare needs and identification of ways in which services should be improved
> - Are an essential starting point for planning any changes to services or interventions

Project design

The design of a study refers its overall structure. This structure has to be appropriate to the aim of the project. A wide range of terms can be used to describe the design of a study. Some of the most common design features and their application in pharmacy practice and related projects are outlined here.

Many descriptive studies are *cross-sectional* in that data are collected from the population on one occasion only. Data usually relate to a single point or period in time, providing a snapshot. Most questionnaire studies are cross-sectional. The information requested usually relates to previous, although recent, events (i.e. *retrospective* - relating to what has happened in the past) or concerns the present time or situation. Cross-sectional studies collecting data relating to current situations or events, are also termed *prevalence* studies (i.e. to establish the number of cases of x in a population at a point or period in time). Studies which comprise a descriptive, often frequency, analysis of cross-sectional data are also referred to as *observational studies*. These can be distinguished from observation studies in which a researcher is physically present in a setting, to watch and records events of interest (see **Chapter 11**).

In some studies, respondents are requested to maintain records of events, symptoms, etc. over a period of time (e.g. keep a diary). Thus, the study may be *prospective* (relating to future events). Data collection commences at a point in time and extends for a specified period into the future.

Some studies are described as *exploratory*. These commonly employ qualitative methodology, and/or a mixture of approaches and methods (see further) with the aim of investigating a topic from the perspective of different stakeholders and identifying the issues that are important to them. Sometimes they are also *hypothesis generating*, in that they provide clues about the important factors that may influence the behaviour of individuals, or the success of a service, or explain other phenomena. Any hypothesis might then be tested in a subsequent study with an appropriate experimental design (see below).

A *longitudinal study* follows up a sample of individuals or cases over a period of time. Data will be collected from each individual on more than one occasion. These studies are sometimes called *cohort studies* (i.e. a group or cohort of individuals is followed for a given period), and may be descriptive in that a single population is followed up and their experiences described. Alternatively, the study may follow two or more cohorts and be designed to compare their experiences over a period of time. An example would be a study that followed and compared the careers of cohorts of students from two or more different schools of pharmacy over a period of time.

Defining the study population, identifying a suitable sampling frame and employing appropriate sampling strategies and procedures are fundamental to descriptive studies. It must be clear to whom (or what set of cases) the study findings relate. That an appropriately representative sample has been selected (and taken part) must also be assured, otherwise the data cannot be assumed to provide a valid description of the phenomena under study. These issues of population, sampling and generalisability are discussed further in **Chapter 10**.

Experimental studies are designed to test a hypothesis. Clinical trial design (in particular the *randomised controlled trial* or RCT) falls into this category. The important features of RCT design are specification of eligibility criteria, randomisation of the sample between the experimental and control groups, ensuring that the experience of the two groups is similar except with respect to the intervention, blinding of participants, professionals and researchers (as far as possible) to the allocation between experimental and control groups, and selection of appropriate outcomes measures.

In health service and pharmacy practice research, an experimental design can sometimes be used to assess the impact of a new service or intervention. Experimental design, especially RCT design is often viewed as the 'gold standard'. However, in practice this is often not feasible. For example, to assess the impact of layout or other structural features in community pharmacies, it may not be possible to randomise (or impose structural features upon) already established pharmacies. In an intervention study, ethical considerations may mean that patients should be offered a choice of services. Restricting participation to those that have no preference may confine the research to a small, or non-representative, group. In some studies, blinding will not be possible as participants will necessarily be aware of the group that they are in. In these cases an alternative study design, such as a *quasi-experimental design*, may be employed (see below).

An *intervention study* is designed to assess the impact of a change (i.e. a service development or intervention). The selection of an appropriate study design is essential if the research is to be of value. Baseline and post-intervention data will be required to enable an assessment of whether or not the intervention resulted in any change (*before-and-after design*). To be sure that any change was a direct result of the intervention and not some other factor(s), a control group is also needed. A before-and-after design and a control group are features of an *experimental* or *quasi-experimental design*.

For example, a *before-and-after design* may be employed to evaluate the impact of a drug information service on prescribing. Data relevant to the anticipated effects of the service are collected before the introduction of the service and again after its implementation. The difficulty that this design presents is that you cannot be sure whether or not any change was attributable to the service itself, rather than to other factors (e.g. any retraining, staff changes, or publicity that might have occurred). To address this problem, a more robust design would include a control group, which should be similar in all respects to the group of individuals who are receiving the service (the intervention group), except that they do not experience the drug information service. If changes occurred in the intervention group, but not the control group, they could be attributed to the intervention. If individuals were randomised to either the control or intervention group, this would be an example of experimental design. If randomisation is not possible, individuals in the two groups could be matched (see **Chapter 10**), thus resulting in a *quasi-experimental design*.

The *evaluation* of services will often involve its effects on patient care as well as implications for professionals, patients, health organisations and health policy. All these potential impacts should be taken into account in the design of the evaluation. In addition, service developments are implemented in natural settings (i.e. in the context of a wide variety of healthcare or pharmacy settings, situations and circumstances). To take all these 'real world' factors into account, a *holistic approach* to study design may be desired. This may entail a complex design. The evaluation may comprise a group of studies among the different stakeholders to examine the effectiveness and feasibility from their different perspectives. Separate sampling strategies, methods of data collection, outcome measures, etc. may have to be identified for each group. Thus, such an evaluation may involve a combination of different methodological approaches and the measurement of a wide range of variables relating to aspects of the structures, processes and outcomes of the intervention.

Feasibility studies are often small-scale studies that aim to assess aspects of the efficacy or practicalities of an intervention. They are generally undertaken in a small number of selected settings and often focus on specific features of the service that would be deemed essential for its success (e.g. clinical efficacy or acceptability to health professionals or patients). Carrying out a feasibility study can avoid spending large amounts of money on a randomised controlled trial before understanding key barriers to success and putting in strategies placed to overcome them. The Medical Research Council has suggested a framework for evaluating complex interventions in which it has identified feasibility and piloting of an intervention as a key stage in evaluation. If the feasibility study demonstrates that the service *can work* (albeit in a limited range of settings), it may then be reasonable to extend it to a wider range of situations. A broader evaluation of the service may then follow which asks '*does it work?*' when offered in a typical range of practice settings, under different circumstances, and/or among various patient groups.

A *case-control study* may be hypothesis-generating or hypothesis-testing. These studies aim to identify causative factors or explanatory variables that lead to a particular outcome. Cases that possess the outcome of interest are identified. Each case is matched with one or more controls which are similar in all important respects, except the outcome of interest. Data are then gathered from cases and controls in an attempt to identify factors in the past (i.e. data are retrospective) that distinguish the two groups and therefore may explain the emergence of the observed outcome.

Case-study research focuses on a single or small number of cases in order to examine phenomena of interest. A case may be a setting (e.g. a pharmacy, clinic), single individuals (selected practitioners or community (group meeting of individuals). A mixture of methods and approaches may be applied to examine the operation, events within the setting, and/or the behaviours or individuals.

Process evaluation

In addition to measuring outcomes of an intervention, measuring process can also give very valuable information. This is a measurement of the extent to which the process of the intervention was followed, for example evaluating whether or not training sessions were carried out or posters were put up on a ward as planned. Collecting such information will assist the researcher in interpreting the results of the study. For example, if an intervention has not been successful, process evaluation may help inform the reason for this. Did it fail because the intervention was not fully implemented, or because, although it was implemented, it did not produce the excepted outcomes? This will in turn inform further projects e.g. whether to focus on how to improve implementation of an intervention or developing a different intervention.

Realist evaluation

Realist evaluation is emerging as an alternative design to the randomised controlled trial. A realist evaluation does not simply seek to answer the question of whether or not an intervention works, but rather asks for whom does it work, and under which circumstances. A realist evaluation will begin with a programme theory. A programme theory explains how an intervention is expected to produce the intended outcomes. A series of context-mechanism-outcome (CMO) configurations will then be created. A CMO is the mechanism by which an intervention is expected to affect outcomes in a specific context. These will be tested in the evaluation.

Quality improvement

Another commonly used methodology in pharmacy-based projects is quality improvement, which is the systematic improvement of healthcare delivery. Quality improvement works on the basis of Plan-Do-Study-Act cycles. These involve developing an improvement plan, implementing it on a small scale, analysing its effects and either modifying it or rolling it out further (*Figure 9.1*).

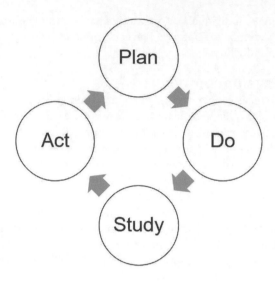

Figure 9.1: *The quality improvement cycle*

The advantage of quality improvement is it provides the tools to evaluate the processes and outcomes throughout a study, rather than only at the end. Baseline data on process and outcome measures are collected at 12-20 points in time, e.g. weekly for 12-20 weeks, before an intervention is put in place. Results are plotted on run charts or statistical process charts, alongside timings of intervention implementation or other events. These are then interpreted to determine whether there have been any changes to processes and outcomes over time. The intervention can then be adjusted if needed, and its effects measured again.

Incorporating theoretical frameworks

Theories provide a way of viewing or explaining phenomena. Researchers from many disciplines have developed and tested theories to explain the operation of organisations, professionalism, illness behaviours including their use of medicines, or how, why and when people engage in lifestyle changes. For example, studies have drawn on psychological theories of how people's perceptions of health and beliefs about medicines influence the decisions they make about taking medicines; sociological theories highlight social, economic and cultural factors that affect health behaviours. In the evaluation of health services, many studies have drawn on a conceptual framework that involves the independent assessment of their structures, processes and outcomes.

Research can be greatly enhanced in terms of its science, scholarship and value when informed by established theories or conceptual frameworks.

When a study is conceived in terms of applying or building upon an established conceptual or theoretical framework, this will be an important consideration in its design. It may also lead to specific requirements regarding, for example, the setting of the study, sampling strategies, selection of measures and methods for data collection.

Pilot studies

Pilot studies (*Box 9.3*) are small studies that are designed to test the methods, procedures, instruments and documentation for a larger study. Before embarking on a large-scale project, it is important to check that the project is feasible and will provide the information required to answer the research question.

Box 9.3: The purpose of a pilot study

This is twofold:
- To check that the methods and procedures are acceptable and feasible in the settings
- To ensure that the chosen methods provide the data required (in terms of completeness, reliability and validity) to meet the study objectives

---

After the pilot study you can review and modify the methods, procedures, instruments or other documentation. You might ask the following questions:
- In relation to the acceptability of the process:
  - Were the recruitment rates good enough?
  - Were sufficient numbers of people/cases eligible?
  - Were people prepared to take part?
- Did you obtain all the information that would be needed to meet the study objectives?
- With regard to the analysis of an existing database:
  - Did you have access to all the data that you needed?
  - Were there sufficient cases?
  - What was the extent of missing data?
- If observing activities:
  - Could you be sufficiently discreet?
  - Did you find that your presence was a hindrance to others?
  - Was it possible to find a private area for interviewing?

When analysing the data from a pilot study you may assess the adequacy of the data obtained for each study objective. You may examine the reliability of data, or any indicators of their accuracy. In a questionnaire or interview schedule you may look for inconsistencies in responses that may suggest ambiguity in the questions. Missing data may suggest that respondents had difficulty answering some questions or did not wish to do so.

The results of the pilot study may lead you to make some changes to the study procedures. For example, to:

- modify the recruitment procedures, e.g. information provided to potential participants, or change the location of recruitment
- reduce or extend a period of observation
- amend an interview schedule, e.g. question order, reduce the length of an interview, etc.
- rephrase questions in a questionnaire to ensure clarity
- modify the layout of data collection from an observation study
- include additional questions on certain topics and/or omit others.

Even though the data obtained in the pilot work will not usually be included in the dataset for the main study, you should keep notes of the methods and procedures used, along with details of, and reasons for, any modifications made to the main study. Details of the pilot study should be included in the project report.

Quantitative and qualitative approaches and study design

Whilst quantitative and qualitative methods may be applied in the context of a range of research designs, these approaches are sometimes associated with particular types of study. Quantitative methods are the basis of large descriptive studies, such as population surveys, as well as experimental studies, which quantify associations between variables or differences between groups.

Qualitative research is most often descriptive, and/or exploratory. It may also be 'theory-building' or hypothesis-generating. These methods are generally only employed in a limited and specialised way in experimental work. For example, this may be to examine contextual issues, and/or enable more detailed examination of potential explanatory factors, relating to the study findings. When a holistic approach is taken to the evaluation of an intervention, qualitative techniques may often be applied in combination with quantitative assessments. For example qualitative data may provide explanation for the quantitative findings.

Triangulation

Many studies combine different approaches, methods, and/or data within a single research study. This is referred to as 'triangulation' (*Box 9.4*). The term triangulation derives from navigation, in which measurements from different positions enable more reliable estimates to be made. Thus, a common application of triangulation in health services and pharmacy research is to validate data. For example, data on pharmacy services may be collected by questionnaire or by observation. In terms of the reliability of information, each would have advantages and disadvantages. Collecting information in two different ways may allow a more accurate assessment. Information from patients on their use of medicines could be compared with data from medical notes or dispensing records. Again, combining data from different sources would enable some assessment of the likely accuracy of information.

Sometimes a study may have both a qualitative and quantitative stage. As mentioned in **Chapter 7** combining qualitative and quantitative approaches within a study is regarded by some as controversial. However, in health services and related research it is not uncommon. A study may commence with an exploratory, or qualitative, stage to uncover and explain relevant issues prior to the development and execution of a large quantitative study to examine these phenomena in a wider, representative population. Alternatively, a survey may enable the identification of individuals who have had particular experiences, from whom more detail could subsequently be obtained using a different approach.

Box 9.4: Triangulation

In health service research, triangulation is employed to:
- provide different perspectives on a set of issues related to the study aims and objectives
- obtain data on different issues and/or from a range of sources, which are relevant to the aims and objectives of the research
- investigate, or demonstrate, the validity of data (by comparing data on the same variables that have been obtained in different ways).

Conclusion

Selection of the most suitable design, approach and method for a study is vital for meeting its aims and objectives. This chapter has provided an overview of principal design features employed in research into health, medicines use and professional practice.

Questions

1. **Which of the following are features of a randomised controlled trial? (Select all that apply)**
   A: Randomisation
   B: A control group
   C: Qualitative data collection
   D: Outcome measures

2. **What is the essential difference between a cross-sectional and a longitudinal study?**

3. **Name five study designs that may be used in pharmacy practice projects.**

4. **Why would a pilot study be carried out?**

5. **What is triangulation?**

CHAPTER 10

Sources of information, datasets, sampling and recruitment

LEARNING OBJECTIVES

Upon completion of this chapter you should be able to:

- identify a wide range of potential sources of data for pharmacy practice projects
- select appropriate sampling methods and discuss their advantages and disadvantages
- choose a relevant sample size
- identify suitable methods for recruiting participants.

At the start of any project decisions are made about sources of, and access to, data (*Box 10.1*). In pharmacy practice research, because of the wide range of topics and methods, these are many and varied.

> ### Box 10.1: Questions to be asked about sources of data and sampling
>
> - Who/what is my population?
> - What data sources are available?
> - How will I select my cases?
>   - What will be my sampling strategy and procedure?
>   - What procedure will I use to select my participants/cases?
>   - How will I deal with non-response, missing cases/data?

Sources of data

The data refer to the information that you need to answer your research questions. In research in healthcare, medicines use and professional practice, potential sources of information can be diverse. Depending on your study objectives, you may seek data from more than one source. Data sources are commonly distinguished as *primary* and *secondary* (*Box 10.2*). Primary sources are data that are collected specifically for the research study that is being conducted. Secondary sources refer to data that have been collected for another purpose, which may have been for a previous research study, or data that are routinely collected for monitoring practice, or other events and activities. For example, if you were investigating requests for medicines information to a helpline, some information regarding all queries may be maintained. You may be able to interrogate this dataset to achieve your study objectives. However, if you required additional information, e.g. on users' perceptions of the quality of the drug information service, you may have to collect additional data of your own (primary data).

> **Box 10.2: Some sources of data that may be used in healthcare and pharmacy practice research**
>
> - Contacts with individuals:
>   - Pharmacists
>   - Other health professionals or practitioners
>   - Pharmacy clients
>   - Hospital or primary care patients
>   - Members of the public
>   - University students
> - Documentary sources and databases:
>   - Research databases, e.g. General Practice Research Database
>   - Databases established as part of previous research projects
>   - Prescribing data
>   - Dispensing data and patient medication records
>   - Patients' medical records
> - Documentation maintained by service providers, practitioners, healthcare organisations, government departments, professional bodies, etc., e.g. queries to a helpline:
>   - Policy documents and other literary sources

Populations and samples

The *population* is the people, cases, events, etc., that the study is about. It is often impractical and unnecessary to gather information from or about everyone in a population, or every case or event that occurs. Research studies commonly focus on a *sample* of individuals, cases or events drawn from the population.

Studies may involve more than one population group. For example, to examine the success of a new educational tool you may to wish examine it from the perspective of both students and tutors, so you will need to sample from both the 'population' of students and the 'population' of tutors. In examining or evaluating pharmacy services you may need to include representatives of different populations or 'stakeholders'. Each group may require its own sampling strategy and procedure. You may wish to compare data obtained from documents with the views of individuals, and this will require a sample of each.

In a study that will involve a sample of cases/individuals, rather than an entire population, you need to decide on a sampling strategy and then your sampling procedures. Your *sampling strategy* is your approach to identifying the *type* of sample that you need. The *sampling procedure* is how you will go about identifying and selecting individuals or cases.

Sampling strategies

The sampling strategy will depend on the aims of your study (*Box 10.3*). With these in mind, you could ask yourself the following questions. The answers to these will help inform your sampling strategy.

- Do I need a sample that is representative of a wider population?
- Do I need to speak to, or gather information about, people or cases with particular experiences or characteristics?
- If an experimental study, are both intervention and control groups required?

Box 10.3: Common sampling strategies in descriptive studies

- A *representative* sample of individuals or cases: so you can claim that findings will apply to a wider population.
- A *purposive* sample: involves the identification of individuals/ cases that fulfil certain conditions, e.g. share particular experiences or work in specified situations and because of their position or experiences are best placed to give you the information that you require for your study. Purposive samples are common in qualitative studies.
- A *convenience* sample: a group of individuals/cases that are accessible and ready to participate. They may not be representative, but in a pilot study may be very helpful in identifying important issues.

If you wish to draw any generalisations from the findings of a study based on a sample, you need a sampling strategy and procedure that will provide you with a representative sample of individuals or cases. The 'gold standard' for selecting a representative sample is a random sample. A random sample is also called a probability sample. A *simple random sample* is one to which all individuals or cases in the population have an equal chance of being selected. Systematic differences between the sample and the population (usually a result of small sampling fractions and non-random procedures) are referred to as *sampling bias*.

If a scientific (preferably a probability) approach to sampling is adopted in terms of sample size and sampling strategy, the study will provide information that can be generalised or extrapolated to the whole study population (i.e. individuals or cases from which the sample was drawn). The applicability of the findings of a study based on a sample to a wider population is referred to as the *generalisability* or *external validity*.

Small random samples and non-random procedures (including quota samples, snowball samples or convenience samples) may not be representative of the wider population. For some studies, e.g. in preliminary fieldwork or studies to inform the methods of a larger study, this may not matter. Purposive or theoretically informed approaches are commonly used in qualitative studies, for which a small number of individuals with specific expertise or experience may be targeted. In devising your sampling strategy, you may need to specify some inclusion or exclusion criteria. For example, if you are examining the use of medicines by a group of patients, you may require that they are using certain medicines, have a particular diagnosis, fall into a specified age range, and/ or possessing other characteristics. You may decide to exclude individuals with e.g. certain comorbidities, who are newly prescribed their medicines, or currently in a secondary care setting.

Sampling procedures

Once the appropriate sampling strategy has been selected, you can start thinking about the different procedures for selecting your participants or cases (*Box 10.4*).

Box 10.4: Common sampling procedures

- Probability samples:
  - Simple random sample
  - Cluster sample
  - Stratified sample
- Non-probability samples:
  - Quota sample
  - Snowball sample
  - Convenience samples and self-selecting samples
- Purposive/theoretically informed samples

Probability samples

Simple random sampling is the most common and straightforward procedure, but there can be advantages to adopting more complex procedures, such as stratified and cluster sampling, which can also be part of a random sampling process.

Simple random samples

A simple random sample is one into which every member of the population has an equal chance of being included. To select a simple random sample, a list of all members of the population is required. This list is called the *sampling frame*. Everyone on the list is given a number, starting with 1. The size of the sample required must be decided; sometimes this is in the form of a sampling fraction (e.g. 1 in 10 sample). The sample is then selected using randomly generated numbers until the required sample size is reached.

If a sampling frame is available, selecting a simple random sample is a very straightforward procedure. Unless there are practical problems of collecting data from a simple random sample (e.g. interviewing individuals widely dispersed geographically), you should adopt this procedure for quantitative studies as it greatly enhances the generalisability and value of the research.

Stratified samples

A stratified sample is one in which the population is divided into subgroups (or strata) before selection. Stratification is particularly useful for making sure that small samples are representative. If the sample size is small, a simple random sampling procedure may, by chance, result in insufficient individuals/cases from minority groups. By dividing the sample into categories (or strata) before you undertake random selection, you can ensure that all groups are represented. A simple random sampling procedure is then adopted for all strata. The sample is called a *stratified random sample*.

If the sampling frame is stratified, proportionate numbers of individuals in each subgroup can be selected (e.g. 10%). For example, in a study of pharmacy students, you may wish to ensure that individuals from different years of study are similarly represented. In other studies it may be appropriate to sample disproportionately, e.g. in research among pharmacists with different levels of experience or specialisation, the population may include very small numbers in some specialities. To ensure a minimum number from all groups, you may need to select a higher proportion from some strata than others.

Cluster samples

A cluster sample is one in which the sample is drawn from a limited number of study sites (i.e. clustered in particular locations). This is useful for populations spread over a wide geographical area. The area is divided up into locations and data collection concentrated in a random sample of these locations. Restricting the data collection to a smaller number of study sites may mean that you can include more individuals from each of these sites (i.e. data collection will be more efficient). A cluster sample is often drawn in several stages, e.g. to study an aspect of pharmacy services across the country you may decide to focus your study on a number of geographical locations. You may begin by randomly selecting a small number of regions of the country and then smaller localities within each of these regions. This may make the study more manageable than selecting a simple random sample of pharmacies from a national sampling frame.

Stratification is sometimes combined with cluster sampling, e.g. if data collection is going to be concentrated in a small number of geographical areas, you may wish to stratify each location in terms of whether urban or rural, or on the basis of socioeconomic variables. This would ensure that the areas selected were representative in terms of these characteristics.

Sampling frames

Random sampling procedures are facilitated by the availability of a sampling frame. In many countries the names and addresses of registered pharmacies or local medical practitioners will be held by health organisations or professional bodies, and lists of students will be maintained by educational institutions. However, confidentiality and data protection may restrict access to the information by researchers. Comprehensive lists are not available for all populations.

Addressing the difficulties of non-availability of a sampling frame can be time and resource consuming. You may need to construct your own sampling frame or develop an alternative strategy:

- If information (names and addresses of individuals) required for sampling is not in the public domain (as is frequently the case in health services research), you may have to collaborate with health personnel (who have legitimate access to the information) to undertake the sampling and recruitment on your behalf.
- For hospital pharmacists: a sampling frame could be constructed by contacting the hospitals of interest and obtaining information from each of them about the population of interest. The collective list could then form the sampling frame.
- Obtaining a population-based sample is generally difficult and expensive. Some government surveys use address files by post code to select participants.

Non-probability sampling procedures

Sometimes it is not possible to select a truly random sample. This occurs if no sampling frame can be found or constructed. Under these circumstances, a non-random sampling procedure may be considered. The researcher then has to find the best possible procedure to obtain a sample that is as representative as possible of the population. Even though the procedure is not random, the researcher may ensure that it includes representative numbers of men and women, people living in different areas or people of different educational levels, or other features deemed important to the objectives of the study.

Non-random procedures are not ideal for quantitative research. Ensuring that a sample is representative can be problematic: however hard you try, the sampling will be open to some bias. When reporting the study findings, possible bias in the sampling, and its implications, must be addressed. If a non-random sampling procedure is followed, the sample cannot be described as a probability sample. The application of probability statistics may be inappropriate. Great care must be taken before suggesting the wider applicability of the study findings. Examples of non-probability samples include systematic samples, quota samples, membership lists of voluntary organisations and convenience samples.

Systematic sampling is the closest to non-random and involves selecting cases at fixed point intervals. For example, for pharmacy clients, a procedure sometimes adopted to obtain a systematic sample is to select perhaps every fourth, tenth and twentieth person who comes to the pharmacy (depending on the sample size needed). It is important to select people at different times of the day, and perhaps on different days of the week, to ensure that the sample is representative of all clients.

Quota samples have commonly been used in market research. Quota samples in some respects may be representative of the population under study. They include specific numbers of individuals from different age groups, male and female respondents, and individuals from different socioeconomic groups. Thus, the researcher can claim that the sample included people with different personal characteristics, and may feel that they can draw some inferences about the wider population on the basis of the selection procedure, but, because the participants were not randomly selected, the sampling procedure is open to some sampling bias which will have implications for the study findings.

Membership lists of voluntary organisations can sometimes be used as a sampling frame. Although they may include a large number of individuals and provide the scope for a large sample, it must be remembered that these members will be a self-selecting group. They would be expected to share some common backgrounds and/or interests, e.g. members of a self-help group may include disproportionate numbers of individuals who have experienced greater problems in the management of their condition and, in this respect, will not represent the total population sharing their diagnosis.

Convenience samples are those in which the researcher selects individuals who are most accessible and willing to take part. Even though individuals from varied backgrounds may be included, they cannot be assumed to be representative of the study population. However, convenience samples are useful in preliminary fieldwork and some feasibility or pilot studies. In these cases, generalisability is less important because the goal of the researcher is often to assess the feasibility of the methodology. Otherwise convenience samples should be used only if there is no way of obtaining a more representative sample.

A *self-selecting sample* is one in which people choose to take part. Self-selecting samples are likely to include people with a special interest in the topic area, and who are therefore also likely to be unrepresentative of the population as a whole.

An element of self-selection colours many sampling procedures. Even when a random sampling procedure is followed, participants who agree to take part will be self-selecting. This is referred to as *response bias* (see further) and it presents similar difficulties with regard to representativeness as sampling bias.

Purposive samples

Purposive sampling is common in qualitative studies. Purposive sampling is a non-random procedure. Its scientific validity rests on the basis that it is *theoretically informed*. A purposive, or theoretically informed, sample is one for which the researcher has preconceived ideas about the required characteristics of the sample. These are based on the aims and objectives of the study, along with established theories about relevant explanatory variables identified in earlier research. On this basis, the researcher makes informed decisions about the individuals or cases that would be expected to be the most effective and informative in meeting the study objectives. Thus, the researcher *purposively* identifies and selects those individuals or cases. This may be targeting individuals who have had particular experiences or high- or low-level involvement with a particular programme, are influential in decision making about service development, or cases for which specific problems, successes or other features have been documented. Although small and non-random, a purposive sample is not a convenience sample. The sampling strategy in terms of the theoretical rationale and the selection procedure must be clearly described and convincingly justified by the researcher.

Snowball sampling is a technique that has been used to recruit members of an otherwise inaccessible, and usually small, population. The principle is that one member of a population is identified and recruited and further participants are contacted through the network of this individual. This is clearly open to serious bias, but the technique may be justified in situations when there is no other way of accessing a population to investigate important healthcare issues.

Experimental and intervention studies

Experimental design

When sampling for experimental or intervention studies, many of the principles of random selection still apply. However, as a result of the design of the study, there are additional considerations.

The design of an experimental study will generally include both an intervention and a control group. If possible, individuals should be randomly assigned to one or other of these groups, as in a clinical trial. However, in health services research this is not always possible, e.g. in many cases people must be allowed to choose between service options or the type of therapy that they want. They cannot just be assigned to receive a particular type of care irrespective of their preferences. To address this difficulty, a quasi-experimental design may be used in which random allocation is replaced by matching in an attempt to achieve equivalence between the two groups. *Matching* involves identification of the important characteristics of the individuals or setting that are believed to be associated with study outcomes. Then, for each participant in the intervention group, an individual displaying similar characteristics is identified and recruited to the control group. Thus, participants in the intervention and control groups are matched on the variables of importance.

Matching is not as good as random allocation because there may be factors distinguishing individuals in the intervention group from the control group that have not been identified or cannot be matched for. However, it is a common technique and may be the best option when random allocation to intervention and control groups is not possible.

Sampling for evaluation studies not employing an experimental design

In the evaluation of many health and pharmacy service developments, a range of approaches can be employed. As many health service interventions have implications for health authorities, health professionals, patients and others, representatives of all these groups may be included in the evaluation. For example, the success of the new service may be measured in terms of its prespecified objectives, and/or the anticipated and unanticipated outcomes, benefits, costs, etc., from the perspectives of different stakeholders. When a holistic approach is taken a range of sampling strategies may be required. These may depend on the availability of suitable sampling frames for each population group. Thus, within a study, different approaches may be required for the selection of patients and health professionals, or for health professionals in primary and secondary care. However, in all cases, the principles of either probability or purposive sampling should be followed if possible.

Sampling and documentary sources

If the information required to meet the study objectives is available from an existing dataset, then the most efficient approach may be to use this. Some studies are based on the analysis of existing databases that are maintained for research purposes. The General Practice Research Database and The Health Improvement Network (THIN) database are widely used in the UK. Other studies comprise a secondary analysis of data that have been collected for a previous study. Data that are routinely maintained for other purposes can also be a useful source of data, e.g. prescribing information maintained by health organisations or hospital pharmacies; electronic medication records, records maintained by practitioners, documentation relating to medication errors or requests for drug information and data maintained by educational institutions. A study may be an analysis of other written or electronic documents (e.g. drug policy guidelines and medicines information available to consumers). When relying on existing datasets as a source of data, decisions have to be made about their suitability for achieving the study objectives (see **Chapter 14**).

In the analysis of databases, it is common to include all eligible cases in the analysis. Where omissions have to be made because of missing data, the researcher should reflect on the possible importance of this and whether it could lead to some bias in the study findings.

In the selection of material from existing datasets, similar principles should be applied as for sampling in other types of study. For example, if investigating prescribing patterns, the data extracted should be representative of prescribers with different characteristics, in different geographical areas or healthcare settings, etc. If examining medicines information available to consumers, the sampling of documents must take into account the full range of sources relevant to the study objectives. If the number and range of potential documents are vast, then a sampling strategy may have to be devised; you may decide to select material from particular sources, reported within specified time frames or relating to particular events. For a study of the content of pharmacy programmes across different universities you may apply stratification so that you have representation of schools from diverse countries, regions or with particular features.

In research into policy in which the principal source of data is written policy documents, a purposive approach to the identification and sampling of documents may be appropriate. It will be important to ensure that you have identified the major channels through which policy is developed, discussed and communicated. This information can then be used to guide a purposive approach, which will ensure that the focus is on those documents most relevant and important to the research objectives.

Literature sources can be a source of secondary data. In such studies, a systematic and informed approach needs to be taken to the identification and selection of material (see **Chapter 8** and **Chapter 14**).

Sampling for focus groups

Focus groups are a useful method of gathering information from people who have some shared experiences or interests. They are commonly viewed as a qualitative research method. The principles of sampling used in other qualitative work will apply. This may be a purposive (or representative) approach for which you have informed ideas about the characteristics or experiences of the individuals whom you wish to recruit. For example, this may be people whom you know hold particular views, practitioners who work in certain environments, students who have followed a particular programme of study, or patients who share particular health experiences. For some studies you may wish to select a representative sample of individuals who fulfil the eligibility criteria for your study.

Visiting groups of people who already meet together or convening your own groups

If groups of people who meet your eligibility criteria already meet together, you may be able to go along to one of their meetings to run a focus group discussion. This can make your life easier than trying to identify individuals, get their agreement to taking part and then making all arrangements at a time that is convenient for everyone, as well as a suitable location and environment for the focus group discussion. Arranging to attend a meeting often requires communication with only one group member rather than all, although this individual may wish to seek the views and agreement from others. In established groups the members will usually know each other and will be aware that they share common interests or experiences, which will be the reason for them attending the group. This may provide the researcher with an opportunity to explore issues with a group who are in a familiar environment and possibly relaxed in each other's company. This may be advantageous to the depth of discussion. As with all groups, the discussion will be coloured by established group dynamics and relationships. Sometimes, in groups in which people know each other they may be less inclined to share certain views than in groups in which they feel anonymous.

Members of special interest groups are, of course, self-selecting. It may be that whilst sharing experiences and views that are relevant to your research, they are unrepresentative of the wider population of potential participants in other ways. For example, they may all live in a particular location or have common social backgrounds.

By convening the groups yourself (i.e. selecting each individual) you are able to ensure some degree of representativeness of the participants. Also, you can often have more control over the number of participants, the location of the meeting and the layout of the room, making sure that it is conducive to a constructive group discussion. Depending on the recruitment procedures and setting, the individual participants may or may not know each other. The contributions of the participants will still be influenced by group dynamics. All groups inevitably include both more dominant and quieter participants.

Numbers of groups and participants

The number of groups required depends on the purpose of the study. Focus groups are sometimes used in the early stages of a research project to identify relevant issues that will then be addressed in more detail in a larger study; one or two groups may be sufficient for this. In other studies, the minimum number of groups may be determined by the need to include a range of population groups.

The number of participants in a group is known to be an important influence on how effective it is. As group size increases, the number of quiet or non-contributing members tends to rise and it is much more difficult for the facilitator to encourage all members to take part. Large groups may hinder the development of an in-depth discussion that focuses on a single topic. However, because there are a larger number of participants, a wider range of issues may be raised. Optimum group size is generally considered to be six to eight participants.

Sample size

The statistical approach to determining the required sample size in quantitative studies is to perform a power calculation. In experimental studies this is based on estimates of the differences in important variables between groups. For a given sample size and level of statistical significance, it provides a measure of the likelihood that a difference between groups will be detected.

In survey research, the sample size required is determined by the degree of accuracy desired when the estimate based on the sample is applied to the wider population. In general, the larger the sample size the more accurate the estimates (and the narrower the confidence intervals) will be. If subgroup analyses are to be performed, it is also important to ensure that there will be sufficient numbers of cases in each subgroup. In deciding the sample size, the anticipated response rate must also be taken into account.

Power calculations and determination of an appropriate sample size can be complicated, depending on the design of the study, the aims of the research and the outcome measures. In many projects, practical considerations, in particular time and resource constraints, also have to be considered. Advice from a statistician may be required.

It is important to remember that increasing the sample size will not address the problem of *sampling bias* (non-representativeness resulting from non-random sampling procedures), although *sampling error* (random error that results from a small sampling fraction) will be reduced. Also, an increase in the sample size will not compensate for non-representativeness that is a consequence of a poor response rate (i.e. response bias).

In qualitative studies sample sizes tend to be small. The objectives of qualitative work are generally served by detailed investigation or purposively selected cases, often adopting a holistic approach. Thus, small samples are often necessary because the work commonly results in vast amounts of textual data. Sample sizes are sometimes informed by previous work, which provides some insights into range of issues and perspectives that are likely to be raised by respondents and the anticipated variation in their experiences and views. This can provide a general indication to researchers of the probable sample size that will be appropriate. *Saturation sampling* is often employed in qualitative research. In this technique, sampling (and data collection) continues until no new topics and perspectives are arising. It is then assumed that the goal of identifying all issues, and perspectives on these, have been identified and sufficient detail has been obtained to enable a qualitative analysis. When saturation sampling is employed, sampling, data collection and analysis can be an iterative process, in that the findings based on the analysis of early cases inform decisions about the selection of further individuals. This may continue until 'saturation' is achieved and/or new issues that have come to light in the course of the study have been addressed.

Recruiting participants in primary research

If you are conducting a study in which you will be collecting data from participants yourself, i.e. primary data, you have to decide on your recruitment procedures, i.e. how you are going to contact your potential participants and make arrangements for the data collection. The recruitment procedures will, to some extent, depend on the type of study and data collection methods. For example, if you are planning a survey by questionnaire, you may decide that a covering letter with the questionnaire is all that is required. If potential respondents are on a single study site, you may decide to hand deliver (and collect) questionnaires. Personal contact may help to promote a good response rate. To maximise response rates it is usual to send out reminders (often two), possibly with a further questionnaire at appropriate time intervals (e.g. 3 weeks apart). It is also good to target potential respondents at a time they are less likely to be busy and involved in other activities. For example, asking patients to complete questionnaires in waiting rooms, particularly where they are there for a prolonged period, can be very effective in maximising response rates.

Questionnaires should be coded so that non-responders can be identified for reminders, and/or in the case of persistent non-response, for follow-up.

This is important. Omitting these codes (to provide anonymity) has not been shown to lead to an increase in response rates. In addition, inability to assess the implications of non-response for the study findings is a shortcoming that can seriously affect the value of the research. Knowledge of the respondents also allows the researcher to acknowledge receipt and thank respondents for their participation.

Invitations to take part in a study and questionnaires are sometimes forwarded by email, either for online completion or return by other means. This requires a list of email addresses of all eligible participants, which will form the sampling frame. Possible concerns about sampling and response are that some potential respondents may not be regular users of email or the internet. Also, for people who receive many messages, if contacts appear casual there is the possibility of oversight of messages and high rates of non-response. However, for some population groups, for whom addresses are available and whose commitment to the study is likely to be high, this may be an effective, efficient and preferred method of recruitment.

A study in which data will be collected in face-to-face interviews will require invitation letters and information to be forwarded and agreement obtained before arrangements for the actual interviews are made. Potential participants may be invited to an interview by the researcher, by a third party (e.g. a health professional) by email, via social media or by post. If researchers undertake the recruitment, they can be sure that procedures are followed and that details of non-response or declines are noted. However, to preserve confidentiality the initial contact may have to come from a professional with legitimate access to records.

Recruitment via social media, such as Facebook and Twitter, has the advantage of enabling access to large sections of the population and may be particularly useful if you wish to recruit participants who use health technologies. However, samples obtained in this way are very unlikely to be limited. The full sampling frame may be unknown.

One of the biggest threats to the external validity of research is non-response. Thus, in devising the recruitment procedures (*Box 10.5*), maximising participation rates must be on the researcher's mind.

Box 10.5: Recruitment and contacts with prospective participants

- How will initial contact be made and by whom?
- What information will be provided in the initial contact, e.g. letters of invitation, information leaflets, consent forms?
- Once agreement is obtained, how will individuals be followed up to arrange for the data collection (distribution and return of questionnaires, arrangements of interviews, setting up of focus group discussions, observation of events)?
- Will it be possible to maintain information on non-responders or people who do not take part, e.g. non-responders may be more common in particular locations?
- How and when will non-responders be followed up with reminders?
- What other steps will you take to maximise response rates?
- After completion of the study will you send a 'thank you' message?
- Will you send a summary of the findings to participants who express an interest?

An invitation letter

A letter of invitation is usually sent to all potential participants. This letter should be as concise as possible and well presented. It should be carefully constructed so that information is in a logical order, easy to read and with all the points clearly made. The letter should inform potential participants of the following:

- The purposes (or aims and objectives) of the research, and why it is important
- How and why they have been selected to take part
- What it will involve for them (what they are being asked to do or agree to)
- By whom the research is being conducted, including collaborators and funding bodies
- That confidentiality will be maintained and that no one will be identifiable in the results of the study (if this is the case)
- Details relating to approval by the relevant ethics committees or other bodies
- Whom to contact for further information

In a questionnaire survey, a copy of the questionnaire can also be forwarded with the invitation letter. For studies requesting personal contact with respondents, visits to premises or access to data, the invitation letter may also include an information leaflet providing more detail about the study. Reply forms for people to indicate if they would like to take part may also be included. For interview studies, it is often emphasised that the interview will be conducted at a time convenient for the interviewee.

Information leaflets

The general rules for the invitation letter apply also to information leaflets: concise information, clear layout and attractive presentation. It is important that it is clear to people what the study will entail for them, including how much of their time you will take and what you are asking them to do. The use of subheadings may be helpful. The content is likely to be similar to that of the covering letter, but it will include further details regarding study procedures, how information will be used and stored, who will have access, a statement about rights to withdraw without care being affected and the procedure should someone wish to make a complaint.

Response rates and non-responders

One of the biggest problems for researchers is non-response. Any response rate below 100% opens up the study to response bias. Many researchers have demonstrated that non-responders are likely to differ from responders in important ways and that this results in bias in the study findings. Maximising response rates and addressing non-response must be seen as an important part of any project.

Response rates of, or near, 100% are rare. They are generally achieved only in 'captive' populations when the researcher is on site, or when potential participants feel obliged to take part (which suggests an ethical problem). Response rates vary dramatically. When high response rates are not achieved (whatever strategy was used in the sample selection), the sample must be viewed as self-selecting (i.e. of doubtful representativeness with regard to the population). This potentially undermines the scientific validity of the work, e.g. it is likely that, in any study, people with a particular interest in the research area would be more likely to respond, and in this they will differ from non-responders.

For researchers there are two important issues. The importance of these cannot be underestimated. They will require time and effort. They are:

- maximising the response rate, to reduce the level of response bias (an important consideration when devising recruitment procedures)
- assessing the impact of the response bias on the study findings.

Maximising response rates

Poor response rates are a big threat to the validity of any study. Steps to achieve as high a response rate as possible must be a priority. Possible reasons why people may be reluctant should be considered in advance

(*Box 10.6*). These can then be addressed during recruitment. Steps taken to maximise response rates should also be described when writing up the project.

Box 10.6: Reasons why potential participants may not respond

- They may not view the topic that you are researching as important. The purposes of the work, drawing out its ultimate value, should be explained.
- They may be unclear about what the study will involve and/or how the results might be used. Make sure that these issues are explained in the initial contact (covering letter, information leaflet or telephone conversation). Be prepared to answer all questions to allay any suspicions. Sources of funding, who is conducting the work and the motives for undertaking it should be stated.
- They may believe that they will have little to contribute. Explain the sampling procedures and the need for representativeness if the results are to be valid. Stress that all contributions are equally important. It should be clear that you have no prior expectations.
- They may be very busy and perceive that the study may interfere with normal working. Researchers should ensure that questionnaires/interviews are as concise as possible. The layout should be attractive and easy to follow; realistic estimates of the anticipated time involved should be given. Payment for time (and/or other expenses) could be considered. At the outset you should consider if what you are asking participants to do is reasonable. Methods that require minimal input or inconvenience on the part of the participant should be devised.
- They may be concerned about confidentiality. In the covering letter and information leaflet assurances should be given that data will be treated confidentially, that no one will be identifiable in the results and that the study has met accepted ethical standards.

Assessing the impact of the response bias on study findings

Non-responders should be followed up to establish how they differ from responders. Some information on non-responders may be apparent from the sampling frame. However, this is generally restricted to a few personal or workplace characteristics, e.g. gender, geographical location, whether pharmacists are from independent, small or large pharmacies, and whether medical practitioners are in single-handed or multiple practices. This information, although worth reporting, may not be of major significance for the research findings. Information on variables important to the research may be established only by direct communication (e.g. by telephone) with a sample (preferably random) of non-responders. Only limited information can generally be obtained at this time, so this investigation should focus on a few key variables that are pertinent to the study objectives. These data can then be taken into account in the analysis and interpretation of the findings.

An alternative approach that has sometimes been used in survey research is to compare the data obtained from early and late responders, i.e. received in response to the first and final mailings. The basis of this approach is that variation between early and late responders may reflect differences between responders and non-responders, i.e. non-responders would be expected to be more similar to late responders. If this analysis is to be conducted, the time of receipt of each questionnaire must be noted.

Conclusion

Sources of data in health services, pharmacy practice and related research are many and varied. For any study there are likely to be alternative strategies and procedures. However, a scientific approach should be applied to both primary and secondary sources of data. For research involving individuals, effective and sensitive recruitment procedures are essential. In devising the sampling and recruitment procedures, researchers need to be mindful of potential problems of insufficient or incomplete data, missing cases, and sampling and response bias. Some assessment of their extent and implications for study findings should be considered.

Questions

1. How are primary and secondary sources of data distinguished?

2. Which of the following are random probability samples? (Select all that apply)
    A: You pick the first 15 male and 15 female pharmacy students in your year who respond to an email inviting them to participate in your study
    B: You divide the pharmacy students in your year into those under 25 and those over 25. You then use randomised numbers to select 15 in each of these groups
    C: You use randomised numbers to select two schools of pharmacy in the UK. You then sample all final year students in these two schools
    D: You put the pharmacy students in your year in alphabetical order and select every fifth student

3. What is a sampling frame?

4. What factors should be considered when identifying a sample size for a study?

5. Identify at least two data sources or recruitment methods you could use for your study to meet your aims and objectives. What are the advantages and disadvantages of using these methods?

CHAPTER 11

Data collection - survey research and questionnaires

LEARNING OBJECTIVES

Upon completion of this chapter you should be able to:

- describe the steps in constructing a good questionnaire
- discuss the advantages and disadvantages of different methods of questionnaire distribution
- describe different types of reliability and validity in relation to research using questionnaires.

Survey research using questionnaires is the most common method in pharmacy practice research. It is used in a wide range of different studies. Questionnaire research is often viewed as a very straightforward approach. However, there are many challenges in ensuring that it is scientific.

Questionnaires can be very useful for collecting information from large samples relatively cheaply, and generally in a reasonably short time. However, these perceived advantages can detract from the potential challenges that scientifically robust questionnaire research presents. The time required can easily be underestimated. Devoting sufficient time to developing and validating the instrument is vital if the data are to be useful. Obtaining a sampling frame is not always straightforward. It is usual to send two reminders (e.g. 3 weeks apart), and additional time will be absorbed in waiting for the return of completed questionnaires. Time should be dedicated to the follow-up of non-responders - thus the time for data collection may be quite extended. You should plan your work so that while you are waiting for responses you can be coding questionnaires already received, setting up your database, and/or writing up your literature review. Whilst you may be tempted to start your analysis when you have only a small proportion of your responses, it is more efficient to wait until data collection is complete.

The biggest challenge to survey research can be achieving a good response rate. Low response rates (which are not uncommon) can result in serious *response bias*, which can jeopardise the generalisability of the data and the value of the research. Careful thought should be given to how you can maximise your response rate; planning how you will approach and recruit your potential respondents and in the design of your questionnaire. You should also attempt to assess the extent and likely impact of response bias on your findings. You cannot assume that people who choose to respond are representative of the wider population. These issues are discussed in more detail in **Chapter 10**, as they are important for many types of research study.

Costs include administration, postage (for repeated mailings and return of questionnaires), and perhaps telephone follow-up of non-responders. Most questionnaires are designed for self-completion by the respondent. However, they may also be completed in interviews with a researcher; this can increase costs in terms of researcher time but also has some advantages.

Although questionnaires are seen as an efficient method of data collection from large numbers of individuals, this does depend on the type of data required. They are considered good for factual data, but this assumes that people are able to provide the relevant information, e.g. people may have difficulty recalling the last time they visited a pharmacy, how long they have been taking a particular medicine, or the names of medicines that they are currently using. People may be unwilling to provide some information (e.g. relating to personal or business issues), or they may not know the answers to some questions. They may, in an effort to be helpful, guess or provide unreliable responses, or they may be influenced by their perceptions of the purposes of the questionnaire and the researchers' expectations. These potential problems may undermine the reliability and the validity of the data. All these possible problems must be considered when you are developing your questionnaire. *Table 11.1* summarises some of the advantages and disadvantages of questionnaires.

Table 11.1: *Summary of perceived advantages and challenges of questionnaires*

Perceived advantages	Comments and potential challenges
Costs of data collection are low	Administrative costs of preparing questionnaires, address files and envelopes, costs of mailing of questionnaires, reminders and returns
Can collect information from a large number of people	Response rates may be low, and this can be the biggest challenge, especially for postal and internet surveys
Data can be collected in a short period of time	Need to think about time and effort in producing a valid instrument, timing of distribution of the questionnaire, waiting for responses, timing of reminders and follow-up of non-responders
Good for factual information, which requires short answers and closed questions	Questions must be easy for people to understand and answer. There is no opportunity to clarify ambiguous or missing responses or to explore further any interesting issues
Structured questionnaires can collect relevant information in a systematic way	Structured instruments require a lot of preparation to ensure that they are valid and reliable and meet the study objectives

Developing your questionnaire

The questionnaire is referred to as the *research instrument*. Constructing the questionnaire is an important part of a research project. It is worth investing enough time and effort at this stage to ensure that the instrument is scientifically robust, effective in providing the required data, and attractive and easy to complete for respondents. If the questionnaire is poor, this will be reflected in the data obtained and the value of your study. Once the questionnaire has been distributed there is no further opportunity for you to make any improvements: change any questions, revise question structures, add items or correct errors. Conversely, if the instrument has been rigorously prepared, issues of validity and reliability have been fully considered and attention has been paid to the presentation, covering letter, etc., then much of the complex work has been done. The responses will be meaningful, data processing will be straightforward, and the analysis will not be hampered by concerns over the quality of the data.

The next sections provide a guide for developing a questionnaire. This includes the content/coverage of the questions and response options, question structure and (in the case of closed questions) possible responses, types of questions likely to present problems, surveys of views and measuring attitudes, and questionnaire layout and organisation.

Content and coverage of the instrument

The first issue to consider when developing the questionnaire is the content or coverage of the questions, i.e. what information do you need? The *content validity* is concerned with the extent to which all information required for the study objectives is collected. You need to be sure that you are gathering information on all important issues and that the response options (in closed questions) cover the range of views or experiences of your potential respondents. Many people will have had the experience of being sent a questionnaire and feeling that important questions are missed, or, in relation to any question, that none of the possible responses really reflects their experiences or views. This can lead to two problems. Firstly, if respondents try to select the best option, you are not obtaining information on their true experiences. Secondly, if they find it difficult to respond, they may choose to skip the question which results in incomplete questionnaires and missing data.

How to achieve content validity?

The content of your questionnaire will be guided by the study objectives. You need to identify the information that you need for each of your study objectives. Sometimes the information that you require may not be immediately obvious. For example, if you are interested in problems that people have in using their medicines, there may be factors that you have not thought about that are important to some people. You need to make sure that in your preliminary fieldwork or literature review you identify as many of these issues as possible.

Content validity must be achieved from the perspective of your study population. It is not safe, generally, to rely on a list generated by an individual or group of researchers. Thus, an important stage of construction of the questionnaire is preliminary fieldwork to ensure content validity of the instrument. This may take the form of a small number of interviews with key individuals (often representatives of the study population), supported by reviews of the literature. This process enables the identification of all issues relevant to the aims of the study, thus promoting content validity.

In addition to ensuring that the questions cover relevant topics, you must also check the response options. These need to be discriminatory, i.e. pick up relevant differences between individuals. They must also accurately reflect people's real feelings or experiences. Checks on the validity, reliability and sensitivity of the response options should also be done as part of the preliminary fieldwork and/or pilot study.

Question structure

Once the content of the questions has been decided, the next task is to construct the questions. The following are important considerations:
- Open or closed questions
- Objective, subjective or relative quantifiers
- Single or multiple response options
- Avoidance of questions that can be problematic

Questions may be closed or open (Box 11.1)

Box 11.1: Closed and open questions

Closed question
How would you describe your health?

Excellent	☐
Good	☐
Fair	☐
Poor	☐

Open question
How would you describe your health?

_____

_____

_____

_____

_____

Closed questions include a 'stem' followed by a limited range of responses. As discussed above, ensuring that the responses include all the likely answers is an issue of *content validity* that should be addressed in the preliminary fieldwork or pilot work. In addition, the response options should be discrete (no overlap) and mutually exclusive (only one possible answer for each respondent) unless the question is intended to be multiple response (see further).

Closed questions are often preferred in self-completion questionnaires. If well constructed they are quicker and easier for respondents to answer, they generally lead to fewer *missing data*, and they are easier for the researcher to code and incorporate into quantitative analyses.

Open questions are often of less value in self-completion questionnaires. As they take longer to answer and may require more thought, respondents are more likely to leave them out. If they are answered, responses to open questions are often brief, which makes them difficult to interpret. When categorising responses so they can assign a code, researchers often have to make assumptions about the meaning behind a response.

Despite their limited value, researchers often like to include a few open questions so that respondents have the chance to provide unsolicited comments on the research and an opportunity for some freedom of expression in answering. Open questions are commonly included at the end of a questionnaire to allow respondents the chance to add any issues that they feel are important and have not been covered in the questionnaire. This can also be useful as a check on the content validity.

Questions may use objective, subjective or relative quantifiers. Many questionnaires require respondents to estimate the frequency of events or the importance of particular issues.

In estimating the frequency of events respondents may be asked to make an objective assessment based on real time (e.g. daily, at least once a week, etc.) or to estimate the number of cases in which an event or situation has occurred. The data from this type of question (assuming that responses are reasonably accurate) enable the researchers to provide summary information about the actual frequency of events.

Subjective assessments provide a picture of the perceptions of respondents of the frequencies compared with what they may believe to be the norm or an ideal. For example, a question may ask respondents to estimate the frequency of an event as rarely, quite often, very often, etc. It is widely acknowledged that what is seen as frequent by one person, may not be by another. If you ask a question using 'subjective' or 'relative' quantifiers, you will not be able to use the data to provide an estimate of the actual frequency of events. Depending on the objectives of your research, you may wish to establish the actual frequency of an event, or respondents' perceptions. In constructing the questions, the researcher must ask him- or herself whether an objective or a subjective assessment is required (*Box 11.2*).

Box 11.2: Subjective and objective quantifiers

Subjective quantifier
How often do you miss a dose
of your medicines?

Often	☐
Sometimes	☐
Occasionally	☐
Never	☐

Objective quantifier
How often do you miss a dose
of your medicines?

At least once a day	☐
At least once a week	☐
At least once a month	☐
Less often than this	☐

Multiple response questions

Most commonly respondents are asked to select a single response to
each question. Multiple response questions are closed questions in
which respondents can select more than one response. For example,
a respondent may be asked to select their top three preferences from
a given list of possible items, or, they may be asked to list up to three
medicines-related problems that they have experienced. The researcher
must make decisions in advance about how many responses will be
allowed, whether they should be ranked in order of importance, etc. It
must be clear to respondents how the question should be answered. A lack
of clarity in the directions will present problems in the interpretation and
coding of data.

Multiple response questions are generally less straightforward when it
comes to coding and analysis. A clear plan for this should be made when
the questionnaire is being constructed. Researchers should also check,
before they embark on data collection, that the structure of the data
obtained from multiple response questions will enable them to conduct
a meaningful analysis. An alternative approach is to construct separate
questions for each of the response options. Whilst this may lengthen the
questionnaire, it may also result in more manageable data.

Questions that can be problematic

When you are constructing the instrument, it can be very easy to overlook
unclear questions or ones that may present other difficulties and affect the
reliability of data. Another pitfall to avoid is asking questions which may
be judgemental in any way or promote a socially desirable rather than a
true response; for example, 'Are you careless with your medicines?' During
preparation and pilot work you should carefully screen your questionnaire

to identify any potentially problematic questions. It can be very helpful to ask a colleague and others to look at the questionnaire too. You could do this before any formal piloting. If you have any uncertainties about whether or not your questionnaire will give you the information that you need, or you have concerns about whether the information will be dependable, you should do some pilot work. Features of questions that often lead to problems are listed in *Box 11.3*.

Box 11.3: Features to look out for when screening and/or piloting your questionnaire

- Questions for which respondents may have a problem in providing the requested information, i.e. when they do not know the answer, e.g. a pharmacist may not know whether a local surgery has specific policies relating to aspects of prescribing or patient care.
- Questions requiring respondents to recall information, e.g. a person may find it difficult to state when they last spoke to a pharmacist, took a particular medicine, etc.
- Questions requesting sensitive information, e.g. personal or business details that people are not happy to disclose.
- Ambiguous questions that may be interpreted in different ways by different people and therefore lead to unreliable or missing responses.
- Double-barrelled questions (e.g. 'Are your colleagues on the ward friendly and helpful?') to which the researcher assumes a single answer can be given, but when it comes to the analysis cannot be sure to which aspect of the question any response relates.
- Questions that include a negative; it is recognised that these questions are more likely to be misread, so it is sensible to try to keep them to a minimum and to underline the actual negative.

Questionnaire about views and attitudes

Developing a questionnaire to assess attitudes is a complex task. In developing these instruments many years' work is often required to explore and examine the factors and dimensions that are important underlying determinants of an attitude. The researcher then has to construct an instrument that accurately and effectively measures those factors. These instruments need to have a sound conceptual and theoretical foundation; at the same time they must comprise statements that respondents can readily understand and identify with.

Questionnaires to measure attitudes generally ask respondents to give their views on a series of statements. These statements, or questionnaire items, need to cover the range of views and beliefs that reflect the attitudes of individuals on the phenomenon of interest. In addition to establishing the content and breadth of the questionnaire items, the researcher has to think about the depth and strength of feelings in relation to all these components. Thus, for any subject, there may be a wide range of issues that need to be included for a comprehensive picture of people's perspectives. Also, some individuals may also hold very strong views or opinions, whereas others may be less concerned.

It is difficult to demonstrate objectively that the items accurately reflect the relevant components in terms of beliefs, experiences and values. That is, it can be difficult to demonstrate than an instrument possessed both content and construct validity. So, once an instrument has been developed, further work goes into testing it and establishing its validity and reliability. This is a very complex task. Questions that might be asked include the following:

- Is it really a good measure of people's views on a topic?
- Does it enable people with positive and negative views to be distinguished?
- Are the responses to the items reliable?
- As a whole, are the responses of individuals to different items consistent?
- Is it valid for use in different population groups?

Many questionnaires in health services and pharmacy practice research that claim to assess attitudes merely request the respondents' views on a topic. It is better to describe them as a survey of views, opinions or experiences, rather than a measure of attitudes. If a true attitudinal measure is required, if possible, it is best to find an established and validated tool from the literature rather than attempt, in a limited period, to develop one of your own. A similar argument applies to the measurement of health status, quality of life, socioeconomic status, etc., which are also complex constructs (see further).

If you are to embark on the development of a new measure, rigorous fieldwork will be required. Attention must be paid to the content and construct validity (i.e. that all the relevant domains and issues are identified and that items accurately reflect these), that statements represent different strengths of feeling in relation to different issues, to the balance of positive and negative items, etc. As in any questionnaire, all items must be reviewed to avoid potential problems arising from question structure or interpretation. Likert scales (strongly agree, agree, neither agree nor disagree, disagree, strongly disagree) are commonly used for responses to items in these questionnaires. A Likert scale is not a true linear scale, and so caution must be exercised in the use of scores for the individual items. In most instances, the data should be viewed as ordinal or nominal (see **Chapter 15**).

Reliability and validity in questionnaires

Issues of reliability and validity have to be addressed in all research. These general concepts have been discussed in **Chapter 7**. In relation to survey research and questionnaire design, some potential problems have already been raised in the above sections. In the case of questionnaire design:

- Reliability refers to the extent to which the questions produce reproducible responses and/or are internally consistent.

Questions that may produce data that are not reliable include those for which people may have difficulty recalling events, questions for which they may not be sure of the answer, questions which are unclear, ambiguous or complicated. It is important that when developing a questionnaire, each question is screened to check that it does not present difficulties which will mean that you cannot rely on the accuracy of the responses. For some questions, you may be confident of the reliability of data; for example, people usually do not have difficulty in reporting their age, details of recent events, or their involvement in current activities. However, for other questions (e.g. requiring recall of events or precise knowledge) the reliability may need to be established. There are a number of ways in which formal checks on the reliability are done. Collecting data from a subset of respondents on two occasions enables the test-retest reliability to be checked. For some questions, information provided in questionnaires can be checked against another source, e.g. reported medication use against prescription data. This is sometimes referred to as triangulation (see **Chapter 9**). Consistency between responses of individuals to different questions can also be examined.

Validity is a more complex concept. In a scientifically robust study, it needs to be addressed in a systematic way. In relation to questionnaire design:

- Validity refers to the extent to which the questions provide a true measure of what they are designed to measure.

It can be very difficult to demonstrate that a question, or series of questions, in a questionnaire provides an accurate reflection of an individual's views, behaviours or experiences. For example, some respondents may be reluctant to report that they indulge in unhealthy behaviours or do not adhere to health advice. Other variables are very complex to define. Inevitably, problems will arise in constructing questions that provide an accurate and comprehensive measure.

Sometimes questions can provide information that is *reliable* (in that people provide consistent answers) but is of doubtful *validity* (the questions and responses are not a true reflection of the issue that we are trying to measure). You should screen all questions or items in your questionnaire to identify possible problems in their likely validity and reliability. Your steps to identify and address any problems should also be discussed in your project report.

The following section provides an overview of the concept of validity in relation to the development of a questionnaire and some guidance on identifying and addressing potential issues. To aid in this, four 'types' of validity can be distinguished:

- Face validity
- Criterion validity
- Construct validity
- Content validity

Face validity is usually the first check to be made. It addresses the question, without further investigation, i.e. *prima facie* would a question be expected to produce accurate information? Checks on the face validity aim to uncover fairly obvious problems such as spotting ambiguous questions or those that may be expected to lead to inaccurate responses. A face validity check may highlight a poorly worded item or topics which may be important but are not included. A check on the face validity can be carried out by members of a research team including supervisors, other experienced researchers, or interested individuals who are not part of the study but may bring fresh eyes to reviewing the instrument. It may be worth asking a range of people. Together they may provide useful feedback for refining the questionnaire, leading to a more reliable and valid instrument.

For some questions you may believe that problems with reliability or validity are unlikely to arise. This may be because questions are very straightforward, have been used in previous studies, or have been validated by others. The face validity check may be all that is deemed necessary. If you believe this to be the case, when you write up your project report you should justify this viewpoint.

Criterion validity refers to whether or not questions correlate with other measures of the same variable; for example, you may ask people about the medicines that they are prescribed and compare responses with data from records. In a study asking prescribers about their compliance with guidelines, a check may be conducted with data on prescribing patterns. Questionnaires may also be used for diagnostic purposes, which are known to correlate with clinical measures. To address potential concerns about the reliability and validity of measures, it may be possible to compare responses from questionnaires with data collected from other sources.

Construct validity is concerned with the extent to which questions accurately represent a concept or construct. Thus, construct validity applies to complex variables; for example, in research into healthcare and the use of medicines, we often wish to report the socioeconomic status of our respondents - thus, we need questions to establish this. In the UK, social researchers generally focus on occupation. However, questions about education, home ownership, income, lifestyle, etc., are also sometimes used. These questions are assumed to be a valid indicator of what people term 'social class'. Similar problems arise in the measurement of 'health-related quality of life'. Again, people will differ in the aspects of their life that they value and how these relate to their health status. Many measures of quality of life, health-related quality of life and health status have been developed and validated to enable these constructs to be included in survey research with a wide variety of population groups. As discussed in **Chapter 7**, when you are constructing your questionnaire, it is advisable to incorporate established measures of complex variables (where they exist) rather than attempt to develop your own.

Content validity refers to the extent to which data gathered cover all the issues relevant to the study objectives. It refers to the domains or topic areas of any questionnaire as well as, in closed questions, the response options. The response options as discussed above must also reflect the diversity of views and experiences of respondents. An acceptable length for a questionnaire may be something that you want to discuss with potential respondents or other researchers or in the pilot work.

Questionnaire organisation and layout

The presentation, organisation and layout of the questionnaire are important because respondents will use it to judge the quality of the study. In contrast to an interview, in which the respondent may not see the interview schedule, potential respondents will probably look through the questionnaire and make an assessment of its potential value, complexity and the time that will be required. These factors will influence whether or not they complete it. Their first impression about its presentation may be very important.

The questionnaire should be headed with the title of the project, together with a reminder of its principal purpose and the organisation carrying out the research. The print should be easy to read. In its layout, it should be clear and easy to follow. Respondents should not have to waste time working out which questions lead on from which, and where to move on to should a question be 'not applicable'. The question order should be logical, so that the overall questionnaire structure is easily discernible. Some thought should be given to which questions appear first. It is common to place questions relating to personal or professional information (age, sex, working situation, etc.) at the end of the instrument. Towards the end of the questionnaire an opportunity (usually in the form of an open question) for respondents to add any further comments that they believe are relevant can be provided. It is worth remembering that if respondents complete only part of the questionnaire, it is the later sections that are more likely to be missed.

A code (to identify the respondent) should be included at either the top or the bottom of the questionnaire. This enables a follow-up of the non-responders, which is important for the study findings. There is no evidence that omission of a code, which enables identification by the research team but preserves anonymity in data coding and analysis, improves response rates to an extent that enhances the value of the research. However, names, addresses and other potential identifiers should not appear and assurances of confidentially should be provided.

Structured questionnaires may also be pre-coded; that is response codes that will be entered directly into a database may be included in the questionnaire (see **Chapter 15**). This can result in a one-stage process of data processing, as the responses do not have to be coded first. It can also be beneficial in that it requires the researcher to think ahead about question structure and relate this to proposed analytical procedures. Advance planning of the analysis required to achieve the study objectives helps to ensure that questions are appropriately formulated and structured.

Other ways of collecting questionnaire data

Interviews

Many questionnaires that are designed for self-completion can also be used in an interview. In general, interviews are preferable for less structured instruments, which often comprise a higher proportion of open questions. Interviews provide an opportunity to follow up any ambiguous or interesting responses. They also enable some flexibility on the part of the interviewer in responding to, and exploring further, issues raised by the respondent that are deemed relevant to the study objectives. However, interviews are more labour intensive and a large sample size may have to be compromised if they are used as an alternative to self-completion questionnaires. Some data collected in a questionnaire could also be gathered through direct observation by a researcher. This has the advantage of providing data on actual events rather than a respondent's reports of these events. Again, because these studies are labour intensive, a large sample size may not be feasible.

By telephone

Questionnaire data may also be gathered by telephone. In general, telephone interviews are more suited to structured questioning, and of more limited value in qualitative work, although they can afford some opportunity to gather thoughtful and considered responses. They have some advantages over self-completion questionnaires; for example, they may enable data to be collected over a shorter period, rather than waiting for responses to questionnaires to arrive by post, and sometimes have a positive impact on response rates. Telephone interviews can be cheap and efficient means of collecting questionnaire data, although mobile phones can be more costly. In collecting the data, the interviewer can ask for clarification or further detail if necessary, in response to any question. However, sample members must be individually identifiable and contactable by telephone. For landlines, it may be more difficult to verify the status of the person to whom you are speaking. Sometimes the presence of others or a lack of privacy (which the researcher will not be aware of) may affect the frankness of responses.

Telephone interviews have been used successfully in many studies. They should be arranged in advance, so that they are at a time convenient for the interviewee. Advance information about the study may also improve cooperation of the interviewee and lead to a more successful interview.

Internet and email questionnaires

The internet is increasingly used as a means of gathering structured information from individuals. Assuming availability of email addresses of the target population groups and adequate response rates, this may be an efficient means of data collection, and preferred by some respondents. Questionnaires distributed electronically can be completed and returned online or by other means. Sometimes online distribution of questionnaires can precede a telephone interview, which enables a potential respondent to see the questions prior to responding. When developing the instruments, similar considerations about the structure of questions, length of questionnaire, organisation and navigation will apply, as for survey data collected in other ways.

There are several software packages and online tools available for constructing and distributing questionnaires; examples of these are Qualtrics and SurveyMonkey. The advantages of using such tools are a professional appearance and a low level of labour being required in terms of distribution and return of questionnaires and data entry. Disadvantages are that the response rate is generally lower than for face-to-face recruitment and that participants without access to internet or preference for paper-based questionnaires will be less likely to participate.

Conclusion

Questionnaire research is common in health service and pharmacy practice research. It is an effective and efficient means of data collection for many studies, but there are pitfalls. It is worth taking time in the early stages to ensure that the instrument is scientifically rigorous, and will produce data that are of sufficient reliability and completeness to achieve the study objectives. Concerns about the quality of data cannot easily be addressed once data collection is under way. If time is invested in developing an instrument of high quality, the data processing and analysis will usually be straightforward.

Questions

1. **Which one of the following is a test for content validity?**
   A: Measuring against a gold standard to check the degree of association
   B: Testing whether participants give similar responses to questions one week after they first complete the questionnaire
   C: Checking your questions are clear
   D: Checking your questionnaire covers the data that is relevant to the objectives

Try rewriting each of the following questions to improve them.

2. **Did you find that the training was easy to understand and covered relevant content?**

3. **Do you leave medicines in a place that puts your children at risk?**

4. **Which age group do you belong to:**
   A: Under 20
   B: 20-40
   C: 40-60
   D: 60-80
   E: Over 80

5. **Do you take your tablets after dinner?**

CHAPTER 12

Data collection - interviews and focus groups

LEARNING OBJECTIVES

Upon completion of this chapter you should be able to:

- describe the steps involved in developing interview schedules and topic guides
- identify the principal techniques involved in conducting interviews and focus groups
- discuss concepts of validity and reliability in the context of interviews and focus groups.

Different types of interview are employed in health services and pharmacy practice research. Instruments range through the spectrum of highly structured, through semi-structured, to unstructured instruments for use in both quantitative and qualitative studies. Interviewing, especially in qualitative research, is a highly skilled task. It is greatly aided by an effective interview guide. This chapter will discuss the types of interview, development of interview guides and interviewing techniques for both individual, face-to-face interviews and focus groups.

Types of research interview

Research interviews are very commonly employed in studies into healthcare, medicines use and professional practice. They are employed in many different types of research. In particular, they are a principal method of data collection in qualitative studies. Thus, research interviews are commonly distinguished as *structured*, *semi-structured* or *unstructured* (*in-depth*) (*Table 12.1*).

In survey research, interviews are often seen as an alternative means of gathering information from individuals that is more flexible than in a self-completion questionnaire. In general, a structured interview follows a structured questionnaire that differs from a self-completion questionnaire in that it is likely to include more open questions. In self-completion surveys, open questions tend to be of limited value as respondents tend to write a very brief response, or omit them altogether. Open questions are appropriate if data are collected in an interview, as an interviewer who is skilled can ask for clarification or more detail in relation to any question so that the responses are meaningful.

In qualitative interviews, the interview schedule is commonly referred to as an *interview guide* or *topic guide* to reflect the principles and style of *qualitative enquiry*. The interview guide provides only a framework for the interview. The actual direction and content of the interview, in terms of the issues discussed, is determined by the respondent's experiences, views, perceptions, etc. The interviewer does not want to lead the interview but, in relation to different topics and issues, to find out what is important to the person they are interviewing. It is up to interviewers to use their skills to ensure that the interviews fully explore these perspectives rather than being influenced by their own agenda or preconceptions. Thus, the interview is used to explore issues from the perspective of the respondents.

Many research interviews are described as semi-structured. Semi-structured interviews follow an *interview schedule*, which comprises both structured and open questions and draws on principles of qualitative and quantitative approaches. Semi-structured interviews are appropriate for many studies into healthcare and pharmacy practice, and probably are the most widely employed interview approach. They are used in studies which require information on both predetermined, structured measures and a more detailed examination of pertinent views and experiences of respondents. The open questions provide an opportunity to examine the experiences, problems, concerns and priorities of respondents, in context and with their reasoning. Patients' perspectives are increasingly seen as important in informing the future of healthcare. Interviews provide an opportunity to contribute to this research and policy agenda.

Table 12.1: *The structured and unstructured approaches to research interviews*

Structured interviews	Unstructured interviews
Employed in quantitative studies	Employed in qualitative studies
Researcher led	Respondent led
Mainly close questions: predefined response categories (e.g. tick boxes)	Mainly open questions: respondents express own views in their own words
Range of responses predictable	Range of responses unpredictable
Short answers to questions	Responses to questions may be lengthy

The interview schedule or interview/topic guide

The interview schedule or interview/topic guide is the tool or instrument that you use to help you collect all relevant information from the person you are interviewing. In a semi- or unstructured interview, the instrument will not be totally prescriptive in providing the questions. However, you need to ensure that it is as helpful as possible in enabling you to be effective: covering all relevant issues and obtaining sufficient detail on these, and aiding you in observing the principles of qualitative enquiry to gain the perspectives of the interviewee. In constructing your interview guide you need to consider:

- the content: the topic areas to be covered and any prompts
- question structure: open questions, probing questions to gather further detail
- layout and fonts to assist you in navigating.

The content - identifying the topic areas

The interview schedule, as a questionnaire, comprises a series of questions. As with a questionnaire, the topics that you include will be determined by your study objectives. You could begin writing the interview schedule by constructing open questions around each study objective.

Constructing the questions

For each subject to be included in the interview schedule, a series of questions are required. Typically, examination of each topic in the interview schedule will start with one or more *open questions*. To gather further detail on issues and points made by the respondent, the interviewer will often use *probing questions*. If the interviewer requires information on other aspects that have not been raised by the respondent, they may then use *prompts* to obtain this. Sometimes, once the discussion of a topic has been exhausted, *structured questions* may be used to obtain an overall viewpoint, measure or compare data from all respondents.

Open questions

The purpose of qualitative enquiry is to examine a topic from the perspective of the respondents. Thus, in a semi-structured or unstructured interview, a high proportion of the questions will be open. These provide respondents with an opportunity to describe their views and experiences in their own words, according to the issues that are most important to them. The open questions must be carefully worded to ensure that they do not *lead* the respondent to answer in a particular way.

Open questions often require the respondent to 'stop and think' before they respond. If a question appears very general, they may ask for clarification, e.g. 'What do you mean...?'

A rephrasing of some questions in the interview guide that the interviewer can draw on may be helpful.

Probing for more detail

Once the respondent has outlined their views and thoughts on a topic in relation to an open question, the interviewer may move on to probing questions to gather more detail on these views and associated experiences. Typical probing questions may be:

- Would you say more about...?
- Please could you explain...?
- What do you think are the reasons for...?
- Why do you think that...?
- You mentioned your experience of .... Could you tell me more about this?
- You said this made you feel.... Why was that?

Prompts to ask for comments on particular aspects

Sometimes in response to an open question, respondents focus on the particular aspects or experiences that are more important to them. These data are important. However, the researcher may also want respondent to comment on other aspects. For example, if asked for their views on medicines information, respondents may discuss only oral information. The researcher, having gathered data on this topic, may want to request their views and experiences of written information, labels or that from other sources. Thus, they may use prompting questions (often open questions that may be followed up with probing questions) to obtain these data.

Closed questions

In semi-structured interviews, closed questions are sometimes included to provide a summary of the respondent's views. For example, following a series of open questions regarding a respondent's views and experiences on information about their medicines, the researcher may ask a concluding question: 'So overall, how satisfied are you with the information that you received about your medicines? Very satisfied; Partly satisfied; Rather dissatisfied; Very dissatisfied'. In some cases established instruments, e.g. to measure health status, may be used.

Layout and fonts

The interview schedule should be constructed so that it is as helpful as possible to the interviewer in gathering the relevant data in a scientific way. The layout and systematic use of fonts can also assist with this. If data are to be gathered by a number of different interviewers, it will also help to ensure that they all conduct the interview in the same way.

So that the interviewer knows which questions are to be asked of all respondents, and which are to be used as needed to follow up responses, different typefaces in the interview schedule may be helpful, e.g. the following scheme could be used:

- *Instructions to interviewers could be written in italics*
- **Open questions to be asked of all respondents and text to be voiced in all interviews could be printed in bold type**
- Prompts or probing questions to be used as needed could be in normal print

Interviewing techniques

Interviewing in qualitative research is a skilled task. This contrasts with a structured interview where the interviewer reads the preset questions in a questionnaire and records the interviewee's responses following a predetermined framework. In semi-structured and unstructured interviews, the researcher has to observe the principles of 'qualitative enquiry'. The goal is to identify and examine issues that are important to respondents. Thus, before the interview commences the researcher cannot be sure what issues will be raised. During the interview, the interviewer needs to adopt techniques to ensure that all relevant information is identified and examined in sufficient detail, and in a way that reflects the true perspectives of the respondent. The researcher facilitates a process in which interviewees speak their mind and present their views and experiences. The interview guide should have been constructed as an aid for the interviewer in achieving this goal. In conducting an interview, some general rules are given below.

Think about question order and style

Question order matters. Open questions should always come before closed questions on the same issue. If the interviewer begins with questions on specific points, the respondent's thoughts may be channelled to these points to the exclusion of a more wide-ranging exposition of the issues from the respondent's point of view, i.e. the interviewer runs the risk of directing the interview down a particular path. Only when the interviewer believes that the respondent has no more to add in relation to any question should they request comments on specific points that they believe could be important (i.e. use prompts).

Thus, typically the interview schedule will start with an open question requesting a respondent's views or experiences on a particular issue. Subsequent questioning will depend on the response to this open question, e.g. in probing questions the interviewer may request more description of actual events, reasons why particular views are held, their perspectives on how and why any problems arose, how these were or could be addressed, etc., so that comprehensive data relating to the study objectives are obtained.

The interviewer needs to listen very carefully to responses to the open questions. Sometimes respondents may mention a wide range of issues, but only discuss one or two in any depth. The interviewer needs to make a note of all issues raised so that they can go back and request more detail as necessary. They also need to listen to the detail in any response, in case important and relevant information is not included.

Sometimes in an interview, a respondent may answer questions or discuss issues 'out of order'. This may reflect their perceptions about what is important to the study, or their experiences. It may not be appropriate to insist that a respondent follows your question order, but to allow them to describe and explain their experiences in their own way. If some issues are raised, out of order, you will need to ensure that you collect full data. To acknowledge that any issue has already been discussed, when you come to the relevant sections of the schedule you could say: 'We have already discussed some of your thoughts in relation to this question, but do you have anything else to add?'

Avoid leading questions

These are questions which indicate to the respondent that a particular answer is expected. Respondents are more likely to provide the anticipated response or less likely to give a contrary one. When probing for further detail, the interviewer has to construct their questions as they conduct the interview. It is here that it can be very helpful to have a list of non-leading, follow-up (probing) questions in the interview schedule for the interviewer to use as needed.

Pace the interview

Semi-structured and unstructured interviews also require considered responses from the respondent. Thus, it is important that the pace of the interview allows for this. Silences in the interview are often necessary thinking time for when respondents are recalling or reflecting upon past events. Rushing in with further questions risks losing valuable information. It can also result in poor questioning (such as use of leading questions); the interviewer needs thinking time too to construct their questions.

Avoid interrupting the respondent

The goal of an interview is to obtain accurate information on the respondent's perspectives, priorities or concerns relating to an issue. Interrupting respondents may suggest to them that what they have to say is not important. It may interfere with their thought processes, resulting in the loss of relevant data, and may also make them more hesitant to express their views subsequently in the interview.

Make sure that you listen

It is important to *actively* listen so that you identify all the relevant issues raised by the respondent and follow them up. This is vital for the success of the interview. When responding to an open question a respondent may raise a number of relevant issues. However, unless prompted by the interviewer, he or she may not provide detail on all of them. It is important that the interviewer notes all of them and comes back to each in turn for further elucidation before leaving the question.

Some other considerations for a successful interview

Location of interview and personal interaction

For a successful interview, the interviewer and the respondent should be comfortable and settled. For sensitive topics it is helpful if external interruptions are kept to a minimum. It should be apparent from your body language that you are paying attention to responses, interested in their perspectives and sympathetic to their concerns. You should not be, or appear, distracted by other events or activities going on.

Audio recording

Interviews (except structured interviews) are generally audio recorded (with the permission of the respondent) (*Box 12.1*). Audio recording, and subsequent verbatim transcription of data, provides a complete record of the content of the interview. It is a common procedure in qualitative research. It enables an analysis of respondents' perspectives based on what they had to say rather than on an interviewer's summaries or paraphrasing. It allows you to listen and focus on conducting the interview rather than writing. Experience shows that in most studies, most respondents will be agreeable, especially if the reasons for this are carefully explained and assurances of confidentiality are given.

Box 12.1: Asking for permission to record

The following points can be made:
- It ensures that you will not miss out on any detail that may be important.
- For busy health professionals, audio recording may result in a shorter interview and may be a selling point.
- Audio recording also allows the researcher to conduct a more effective interview. The interviewer can concentrate on listening to the respondent and ensuring that additional details and clarification are requested for all relevant issues.
- Assurances of confidentiality must be given. Once data are transcribed the recording should be deleted.

Some notes should still be taken in an audio-recorded interview. Although these will be minimal, they can be an aid in the interviewing process. For example, if a respondent alludes to an event or viewpoint that you believe to be relevant, you may not wish to interrupt them at that point, but instead make a brief note and continue with the discussion. You can then come back to it and request further detail or explanation.

If a respondent does not wish the interview to be audio recorded, this should not be seen as a problem. Hand notes, as detailed as possible, should be taken instead. The interview may take a bit longer and you can explain that you would like to take careful notes of what he or she says. Immediately after the interview, go through the hand notes and clarify any points where detail is limited or that might later appear unclear. In the analysis these data will be useful, although they cannot be quoted as verbatim responses.

To each interview you should take all the necessary audio recording equipment with you, including a digital recorder and spare batteries. At the start, middle and end of the interview, check that it is being successfully recorded. If, after an interview, you discover that there were problems of which you were unaware, make as detailed hand notes as you can, as soon as possible.

Checking your technique

Familiarising yourself with the interview schedule before you attempt any interviews will assist in ensuring that you gather a comprehensive record from the respondent on the subject of study. It will also increase your confidence. If you are not experienced at interviewing, you should conduct a small number of pilot interviews just to develop and check your technique. These interviews should also be audio recorded. You can then play them back and assess your technique (*Box 12.2*).

Box 12.2: Review of your interview technique

Assess the following:

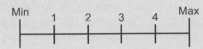

- The use of open questions
- Obtaining additional detail on relevant views and experiences: use of probing questions
- Pacing of the interview and giving the respondent time to consider responses or recall information
- Listening skills: did you 'hear' and follow up all issues raised by respondents?
- Any points or issues raised by respondents for which you should have gathered more information
- Use/avoidance of leading questions
- Unnecessary interruptions
- Taking consent:
  - for participation in the study
  - requesting permission to audio record

Face-to-face or telephone

In qualitative studies, face-to-face interviews are viewed as the norm. However, more structured interviews have been conducted over the telephone. Some advantages are clear in that it may enable a larger number of interviews to be conducted within limited time and resources as they cut out travel time and costs. This is especially the case if the population is spread over a wide geographical area. In some cases, telephone interviews may be effective and justified. However, it is often easier to build a rapport with respondents in a face-to-face interview and to obtain more meaningful, detailed and considered responses. A settled environment, affording privacy and without distractions, cannot be assured in telephone interviews. A face-to-face interview, which will often also be conducted in a natural setting, allows important valuable contextual information to be gathered. This is not possible in a telephone interview. As a consequence of these shortcomings, face-to-face interviews are generally preferred over telephone interviews for qualitative research. If telephone interviews are conducted, telephone recording devices can allow them to be audio recorded.

Reliability and validity in interviews

Potential problems of reliability and validity in interview research must be considered. In a structured interview, many potential problems are similar to those of questionnaires. In qualitative studies there are different considerations. For all interviews, the location can be important; for example, if an interview can be overheard, this may inhibit a respondent from raising and discussing certain issues. Interviewees should be assured about the independence of the researcher and informed of who will, and will not, have access to the data or know what they have said. For your own study you may think of other factors which might be important.

Reliability, which refers to the reproducibility of responses, is in some ways not a pertinent issue in qualitative work. The aim is to examine the relevant issues in context. Any inconsistencies in responses should be followed up in the interview and the reasons for these elicited. It should not be assumed that inconsistent responses are 'incorrect'. Explanations should be sought for apparent contradictions so that a detailed understanding of the issues from the perspective of the interviewee is obtained. Thus, it is important that the interviewer pays careful attention to responses to ensure that all the relevant information is collected during the interview, otherwise difficulties will arise in the data processing and analysis. During the interview process, before moving on to the next question, the interviewer could ask themselves 'Do I have a full understanding of this respondent's view/experience?'

Validity refers to the 'truth' of the data. Some researchers argue that as long as the interviewer is skilled and attentive in observing the principles of qualitative enquiry (i.e. employs a sound interviewing technique), the data will be a true reflection of the respondent's perspectives, and therefore possess some inherent validity. Qualitative data are viewed as valuable because they are a product of the views, priorities, experiences, etc., of people on topics of interest to researchers, practitioners and/or policymakers. However, you must be aware that bias may creep into the data collection process, e.g. by making assumptions about the respondent, or allowing your own preconceived ideas to colour your questioning. It is also important that you are non-leading in the interview and that you can describe the steps that you took to avoid influencing the interviewee in his or her responses.

Reflexivity is a critical reflection by researchers of how their own values or preconceived ideas may influence the process of data collection and analysis. It is especially pertinent to qualitative work where instruments are less structured and there may be more scope for researchers' perspective to creep in. In conducting an interview, it is important for interviewers to be both aware of their own viewpoints or expectations, acknowledging that these could influence the direction of the interview, and also to ensure that they are receptive to the perspectives of the interviewee, even if these do not coincide with their own values and experiences.

Further issues about the reliability and validity of qualitative data that arise in the processing and analysis of data are discussed in **Chapter 15**.

Focus groups/group interviews

Focus groups or group interviews are usually considered a qualitative technique. As with one-to-one interviews, they are conducted by an interviewer, often referred to as the facilitator, who uses an interview schedule or topic guide.

The important difference between one-to-one and group interviews is the interaction between respondents that occurs in focus groups. Thus, commonly, focus groups are employed in exploratory work in which it is believed that the interaction between individuals may stimulate a wide-ranging discussion and generate a comprehensive list of concerns and issues important to respondents. If issues are sensitive, one-to-one interviews may be more effective, if not essential, in providing detailed information. However, if people are prepared to discuss their views and experiences openly, the group setting may provide an opportunity to explore issues raised by respondents from a range of different perspectives (*Table 12.2*).

Focus groups are generally employed in exploratory work, although more structured group techniques, such as nominal group technique, can be valuable. In particular, more structured approaches have been used in consensus building, often involving groups of 'experts' using Delphi techniques.

Table 12.2: *Individual interviews or focus groups*

Individual interviews	Focus groups
More detailed responses from all respondents may be obtained	More wide-ranging discussion may result as participants stimulate each other
May be easier to discuss personal or sensitive issues	May be a reluctance to express opposing viewpoints
Contextual information pertinent to the interview can be collected and examined more effectively	Some participants may tend to dominate the discussion
	Individuals may change viewpoints on hearing the arguments of others
	Group discussion may provide wider perspectives on any issue than would be achieved in an individual interview

Conducting a focus group

A researcher, or facilitator, is responsible for steering the discussion. As for individual interviews, this is done with the aid of a topic guide. The topic guide is usually a semi-structured instrument comprising mainly of open questions with a series of prompts or probing questions to ensure all relevant issues are raised and that all individuals have an opportunity to participate.

The points raised in response to each open question should be fully explored before moving on to subsequent questions. Possible prompts may be:

- Why do you think this situation arises?
- Why do you think people behave/think like this?
- What are the best things about…?
- What are the worst things about…?
- What would you like to change …? How? Why?
- Can you explain that in a bit more detail?
- Is there anything else you'd like to say about this?

Achieving participation of all group members is a particular challenge of focus group research. Inevitably, in any group there will be more and less vocal members. If the facilitator does not plan and adopt strategies and styles of questioning to promote wide participation, the value of group interaction (the reason for choosing this technique in the first place) is lost. It is important to value all contributions, and treat all as equally valid, irrespective of your own viewpoints. In response to each point raised, the facilitator should endeavour to elicit contributions from all participants. When promoting discussion of different views and experiences in relation to each issue, and in encouraging participation of all members of the group, prompting questions in the topic guide may be helpful. For example:

- Does anyone else share this view or have a differing view?
- Has anyone else had a similar experience?
- Has anyone had a different experience?
- Can anyone else describe an example of this?

These questions may then be followed up with prompts for more detail. As with one-to-one qualitative interviews, and for the same reasons, it is usual, with the permission of all participants, to audio record the discussion.

A second researcher (or co-facilitator) is often present. This person does not usually take part in the discussion but ensures the smooth running of the discussion and may take some notes during the discussion to aid the analysis. In particular, it is helpful to be able to distinguish the contributions made by individuals in the transcripts. If contributions cannot be attributed to specific individuals, the extent to which views are shared will be unknown and group interaction, which may be important in interpreting the findings, cannot be taken into account. The co-facilitator should also take responsibility for administrative tasks, operating the recording equipment, organising refreshments, etc., so that the facilitator can concentrate on ensuring an effective discussion.

In terms of the reliability and validity of the data, many of the principles discussed in relation to one-to-one interviews will apply. In focus groups, some individuals may be reluctant to voice opposing views, or those that they feel are less acceptable and/or express the true strength of their feelings, if they feel that their sentiments are not shared. Participants may not wish to raise issues that are sensitive or private. They may be reluctant to share experiences that may reflect on others, especially if they believe that these others may be identifiable. A small number of participants dominating the discussion can also influence the direction and content of the discussion so that the outcome is not representative of the views of all participants. A skilled facilitator will try to encourage views from a wide range of participants.

These difficulties can sometimes be addressed by adopting a more structured approach to the discussion, such as an adaptation of *nominal group technique* or *Delphi process*. To ensure that the views of all individuals are identified, nominal group methods start with a period in which participants silently write out all the views/experiences/thoughts in relation to the topic of discussion. These can then be collated (perhaps anonymously) on a flip chart, grouped together if necessary, and then used to provide the framework for the subsequent discussion. At the end of the meeting, participants could be asked to complete a structured questionnaire indicating their views on important issues or rank the issues identified. This will provide an indication for the researchers of the true extent to which views/experiences that have been discussed are shared by all participants. Whilst primarily viewed as a qualitative approach, various modifications of group interviews have been developed and applied to achieve different goals. The Delphi process involves several rounds of voting in which participants indicate the extent to which they agree with a series of statements. Scores from previous rounds are summarised and included in subsequent rounds. This may be done virtually, rather than face-to-face.

Conclusion

Interviews are a common means of data collection from individuals. Across the spectrum of highly structured interviews (involving administration of a structured questionnaire) to in-depth qualitative studies, they provide a flexible approach that can be employed in different types of study. Conducting qualitative interviews is a highly skilled task. To ensure a scientific approach that accords with the principles of qualitative enquiry, attention must be paid to developing a sound technique. This will help ensure that the findings are dependable and of value.

Questions

1. **Which of the following are open questions? (Select all that apply)**
   A: Did you find it helpful talking to the pharmacist?
   B: To what extent has this intervention had an impact on patient safety?
   C: Has the intervention become embedded in practice?
   D: Do you check the medicines that you are given to make sure they are the right ones?
   E: What are your views on self-administration of medicines?

2. **What are the advantages and disadvantages of conducting focus groups rather than interviews?**

3. **What is nominal group technique?**

4. **What steps can an interviewer take in order to increase the validity of an interview?**

5. **What additional steps can an interviewer take to increase the validity of a focus group discussion?**

CHAPTER 13

Data collection - prospective methods

LEARNING OBJECTIVES

Upon completion of this chapter you should be able to:

- define prospective methods of data collection
- describe a range of methodologies employed in prospective data collection
- identify potential challenges to reliability and validity when using prospective methods and how they can be minimised.

Prospective methods are those in which data are collected as events occur, thus data collection starts at a point in time and extends for a specified period into the future. This chapter focuses on two common approaches: direct observation and diaries.

Observation

In some studies data are collected by a researcher who is physically present at a study site and for the duration of a study period, and observes and records details of events, behaviours or activities as they occur.

In *non-participant observation* the observer is an individual who is independent of the setting (i.e. an outsider). The observer (researcher) aims to be as discrete as possible so as not to interfere with the normal activity. Non-participant observation has been used in qualitative and quantitative studies, but is more usually employed as a quantitative technique. *Participant observation*, in contrast, refers to a method, employed in anthropology, in which the researcher lives or participates as a member of the community or group under study. It involves detailed study of a single community or small number of settings to provide insights into the behaviours, actions and interactions of people in the context of their lives, traditions and situations. These studies are generally qualitative, and methods of observation are commonly combined with interviews and other methods. This technique has been used by researchers examining health beliefs and behaviours, medication use and some aspects of professional practice.

Non-participant observation

In pharmacy practice research, non-participant observation has been employed in many studies and audits. Direct observation has the benefit that data are 'first hand'. They do not rely on individuals' reports of what they do, which may or may not be accurate. Sometimes the best way to collect data on events in real time is to watch what is going on. However, this can present many logistical difficulties and is often not feasible for studies involving large samples. A researcher can only be present on one site at a time. If extended periods of data collection are required, the amount of data that you can collect may be limited. A major concern, and threat to the validity of data, is the 'Hawthorne effect' (see further).

Data collection forms

In quantitative studies, the observer will record details, according to a predetermined schedule, of events or activities as they occur. Often the instrument used will be a structured data collection form, designed for the study, so that for each event or activity similar details are collected. Thus, details recorded will enable an assessment of the frequency of a particular event or activity, the time, its duration, members of staff involved, and other relevant details.

In developing an instrument and study procedures, you need to take steps to ensure that they are effective in gathering the data that you need for your study objectives, and that they are workable (feasible and acceptable) in the study settings. This is best checked out in a pilot study in a few settings which are selected to represent the diversity of locations in which you might be collecting data. This will give you an idea of the number of events that occur, whether or not you are able to collect all the information you need, problems that arise that may affect the completeness or reliability of data, how intrusive/acceptable the procedures are for staff, service users or others, and possible ways of improving the data collection procedures.

Participant observation

Participant observation is a common approach in anthropology. The researcher lives or works as a 'member' of a community to gain insight into and understanding of their situation, beliefs, behaviours, priorities, etc. They aim to achieve an 'insider account' to allow the description and explanation of phenomena from the perspective of the community under study. The researcher seeks to gain their understanding from first-hand experience, rather than as an 'objective onlooker'. This research could be described as holistic, ethnographic and phenomenological. Sources of data and methods may be varied and may include observation, formal and informal interviews and discussions, and documentary or literary sources. Data are commonly collected as field notes. Although not a common technique in pharmacy practice and related research, the work of anthropologists in different parts of the world has provided many insights into different perspectives on health, healthcare and the use of medicines. An understanding of these phenomena in the context of the settings in which they are observed has led many to question assumptions about their own healthcare system and medicines use, rather than to take political, organisational and cultural perspectives for granted.

Anthropologists have in the past typically focused many of their studies in countries where they perceive the culture and traditions to be very different from their own. However there are, perhaps along with the increasing interest in health behaviours and medicines use in social and cultural contexts, examples in which these methods are used in studies within their own populations and communities.

Validity and reliability in observation studies (*Box 13.1*)

When observing and recording activities in any setting, possibly the biggest threat to the validity of the data is the effect of your presence on the individuals you are observing. This is sometimes referred to as the 'Hawthorne effect' after some studies of productivity in a workplace, in which changes to workers' behaviours when they were being observed, masked changes that were a consequence of new working conditions. Changes to behaviour may be conscious or inadvertent. In any observation study it should be assumed that the researcher will have some impact. You should approach the problem in two ways: firstly, consider how you can minimise the Hawthorne effect, and secondly by taking steps to assess its impact.

Possible steps to reduce the impact of your presence may be to explain clearly the purposes of the study so people are not suspicious of your intentions, provide assurances of the confidentiality/anonymity of data, and when collecting data make sure that you are as unobtrusive as possible.

To gather comprehensive data, the researcher needs to be positioned where they can see and (if necessary) hear what is going on. If the researcher is not able to record all relevant details, this will affect the reliability of the data. However, researchers must also be as unobtrusive as possible so that they are not disruptive to those activities that they are there to document. If the presence of the researcher affects normal activities or influences the behaviours of those being observed, this undermines the validity of the data. In most cases the operation of the study and place of the researcher needs careful planning and discussion with staff.

Ideally some attempts should be made to assess the ways in which, and the extent to which, the findings of the study are influenced by the presence of the observer and the research process. Clearly, some activities are more likely to be affected than others. In a pharmacy, an observer may have little influence on the availability on the supply of prescription medicines, but their presence may have an impact on the behaviours of staff. One way to assess impact of the observer is to ask participants at the end of the observation how they felt that the observer's presence changed their behaviour.

In addition, information may be available from other sources (e.g. questionnaires or interviews) to provide some insights into the likely validity of data. Observation itself is also sometimes used to provide some validation of data in other types of studies; for example, self-reporting in questionnaires is sometimes compared with similar information gathered by direct observation.

> **Box 13.1: Questions to ask about the reliability and validity of your data collection**
>
> - Are the events frequent enough so that you will collect sufficient data in the study period?
> - Are the events likely to be (sometimes) too frequent for you to record all details of all events?
> - Is your data collection form precise enough so that you (and others) are clear what information is to be recorded?
> - Can you locate yourself so that you can collect all necessary data in an unobtrusive way?
> - How might your presence affect what is going on? What steps will you take to minimise this?
> - Is there a way that you can assess the effect of your presence on the events, behaviours or other data that you are collecting?
> - If more than one researcher is to be involved in the data collection, can you check the consistency in recording events and the detail obtained?

Other methods of collecting prospective data

Alternative methods of collecting data include self-reports by individuals of events, e.g. in questionnaires, or by requesting individuals to maintain their own records of events or activities, e.g. by keeping a diary. These methods have the advantage that the researcher does not have to be present for long periods in each setting. Particularly for infrequent events, stationing a researcher on site can be unacceptably time-consuming and expensive, especially if an alternative approach can be found. The disadvantage of depending on others to report the frequency of events or maintain diaries is that reliability cannot be assured (see below). In a questionnaire, people's perceptions or memories of events may not be accurate.

Case studies

Case study research is focused around a single case or small group of cases. This may be a particular scenario, an individual, a group of individuals, a single setting, or a set of activities. Case studies may be used to examine behaviours, interactions, activity, events or situations. They aim to capture and document the complexities and dynamics in the context of circumstances and environments, and explain phenomena in the context of their natural setting. Thus, case study research typically draws on qualitative methods, employing an ethnographic and holistic approach. The type of data and methods that will be required will depend on the study objectives. However, in terms of data collection, a combination of methods is often employed so that information on a range of aspects and from differing perspectives can be obtained. Observation, formal or more informal interviews or group discussions, and examination of relevant documentation may all be valuable approaches, providing complementary data and insights.

Diaries

Asking people to keep a diary in which they record details of events or their activities can be a useful method of gathering prospective data. It may be an alternative to direct observation in situations when an observer cannot be present.

Diaries for the reporting of events and activities, and time and motion studies are examples of prospective recording of events. This may be studies involving large samples, when events are unpredictable or rare so that data collection would be time-consuming, or in situations when it is just not feasible for a researcher to be present. For example, you may ask people to keep a diary of their use of particular medicines at home, or ask pharmacists to log discussions with other health professionals during their working day.

Participants recruited to the study are asked to record details of relevant events or their actions. When people are asked to collect data without the researcher being present, questions can arise over data reliability, so steps must be taken to safeguard its quality. In developing your protocol and instruments, you should consider the following:

- The more complicated and labour-intensive the task that participants are asked to undertake, the more likely it is that there will be problems of completeness, reliability and validity. In particular:
  - if events are rare, people can forget that they are supposed to be keeping records
  - if events are frequent and/or at busy times, maintaining records may be impractical
  - if data collection extends over a long period, commitment may wane.
- In planning the study procedures you should consult with potential participants about the feasibility of the task, the likely problems and how these may be minimised. This may help increase their commitment and observance of the study procedures, and realise their importance.
- Data collection forms or diary entries should be quick and easy to complete.
- Limiting time periods of data collection and the level of detail may help increase reliability.
- If instructions are clear, it is more likely that they will be closely followed, which will mean that information is more complete.
- Simple practical steps may make a big difference, such as providing a clipboard for display of the documents, ensuring an appropriate print

size, attaching a pen or, in the case of a diary, discussing the size of the paper or booklet and its layout.

- It is important to check that what you are asking participants to do is acceptable, not too time-consuming or difficult. Study procedures and data quality should be tested in pilot work. During the study, it is a good idea to keep in contact with participants to check whether they are experiencing problems in adhering to the study protocol and to address any difficulties as early as possible.

Time and motion studies and audit

Time and motion studies have been conducted in many practice settings. The methodology employed in these includes structured direct observation and self-reporting of prospective events/activities. The discussion relating to non-participant observation and maintaining of diaries will be relevant to these studies.

Many service evaluations or audit studies also involve observation and/ or the collection of prospective data. Again, attention must be paid to ensuring that data are accurate and representative.

Conclusion

Prospective methods to obtain information on events as they occur can be a powerful technique. Data collection can be slow, especially if the events of interest are relatively infrequent. These studies often require considerable input and commitment by participants. However, because the information relates to real life scenarios, as they occur the information can be more accurate than when relying on their recall. These events can also be examined in relation to their context and setting. Data may also conform to a timeline that provides an opportunity to examine temporal relationships between events, actions and behaviours.

Questions

1. What are prospective methods of data collection?

2. Which of the following are primarily prospective methods? (Select all that apply)
   A: Non-participant observations
   B: Participant observations
   C: Audits of medication administration records
   D: Questionnaires
   E: Diaries

3. Are prospective methods:
   A: Quantitative
   B: Qualitative
   C: Quantitative and/or qualitative

4. What are the disadvantages of using prospective methods in relation to logistics, feasibility, validity and reliability?

5. How might the issues identified in the question above be addressed?

CHAPTER 14

Existing datasets and secondary analyses

LEARNING OBJECTIVES

Upon completion of this chapter you should be able to:

- identify different sources of data for secondary analyses
- describe the advantages of carrying out secondary analyses
- describe potential challenges associated with secondary analyses
- describe different ways of synthesising primary studies when carrying out systematic literature reviews.

Some research questions can be answered by the analysis of data already in existence. If a suitable dataset can be found, this may be the most efficient means of conducting a study. There will be no need to go through a time- and resource-consuming process of collecting your own data.

Sources of existing data are many and varied. Databases that are compiled and maintained for research purposes can be extensive and of very high quality in terms of the comprehensiveness, reliability and validity of the data. Professional bodies, and special interest organisations such as those supporting or representing patients and the public, often maintain records relating to their activities. These can provide useful sources of data for systematic study. Service evaluations and audits often draw on existing, routinely maintained information for the assessment of aspects of professional practice, medicines use and/or patient outcomes.

Literary material and documents are also potential sources of data. Reviews of the peer-reviewed literature, including systematic reviews, meta-analyses of quantitative studies and synthesis of findings from qualitative studies, are examples in which new research questions are examined by bringing together existing data. In some document research, for example policy analysis or the examination of media sources, the documents themselves may be the focus of the study. Content analysis may be performed employing either a quantitative or a qualitative approach.

Working with existing datasets and data quality

When you have not collected the data yourself, you need to be sure that they are of adequate quality for your purposes. You will have had no control over the collection of data and the content of a dataset. You need to make your own assessments of the strengths and weaknesses of the data in meeting your study objectives. You should reflect on these issues when collating and interpreting information and when drawing your conclusions. You should comment on these issues when writing up your project.

Potential problems relating to data quality that you should consider are: comprehensiveness, generalisability, reliability and validity. Difficulties can arise in making these assessments, but you should at least indicate an awareness of possible shortcomings on the dependability of your study findings.

Comprehensiveness of data: Although a database may be huge, it may not include all the variables that you would like to include in your analysis. For example, if you wanted to examine prescribing of particular medicines across patient groups, you may require specific information about patients, diagnoses, medicines, formulations, doses. Are all these variables included?

There may be missing data for cases and variables within the dataset. For example, patient medication records or records of emergency supplies in a pharmacy may be a reliable source for prescription medicines, but less complete for non-prescription medicines. Missing data is likely to be a greater problem for some cases and variables than others. It can undermine the reliability and validity of the analyses.

The dataset may not include a representative sample of the population in which you are interested. It may pertain to certain subgroups, such as those living within a specified geographical area, or certain age groups. This will lead to questions regarding the *generalisability* or *external validity* of the study findings.

Reliability of data: Can you be confident of the reliability of the information that has been entered? Do you have reason to believe that coding and data entry will have been to a high standard? Can you conduct any checks by examining the completeness and consistency of information between or within cases?

Validity of data: What variables are included and how have these been measured? Would the data be expected to provide a true reflection on the phenomena that you are interested in? For example, data relating to adverse effects of a medicine: how have these been verified, recorded and coded?

Established research databases

Some big databases are specifically developed and maintained as a resource for researchers that collate data from many healthcare organisations. For example, the General Practice Research Database contains anonymised medical records of several million patients registered with general medical practitioners in the UK. This is used by pharmacoepidemiologists to examine prescribing patterns and the use of medicines. The Health Improvement Network (THIN) database is another primary care database that may be used for pharmacoepidemiology and other pharmacy practice studies. The Clinical Practice Research Datalink (CPRD) collects data from a network of GP practices across the UK.

Other countries and organisations may also maintain databases relating to the supply of medicines to a population. Some countries maintain a national database of medicines supplied to their population, which may include some anonymised patient information data. Within countries there may be organisations that retain information on their own patients or members. Access to these databases may be restricted, but in some cases, they may be a useful source of information for researchers.

Large population-based health or social surveys, conducted as part of specific research programmes or by government agencies, result in the construction of a database. Once the primary research (the study for which the database was created) has been completed, the dataset may be made available to researchers for secondary analyses. Again, rights and/or costs of access can be restrictive. The value of these databases for answering research questions depends on their content, comprehensiveness and quality of data. They may not contain information on all relevant variables or in sufficient detail. As a consequence, research questions may have to be limited to those that can be addressed by these data. These compromises may impact on the value of the work, but in many instances useful insights and conclusions can be drawn.

Data maintained by organisations

Data relating to their activities are routinely maintained by many organisations. Professional bodies, special interest organisations, as well as those involved in the provision of healthcare may maintain data relating to aspects of medicines use, prescribing and supply, patient monitoring and outcomes, professional practices and procedures, requests for information regarding use of medicines, etc. These data can be a useful and valuable source for research and service evaluation. Additionally, many organisations may be keen for some systematic analysis of their data to be undertaken which may answer important questions about their current activities and help inform future practices. For a study to be of value, it is important that data are sufficiently reliable and complete, and that information extracted is representative of all eligible cases, so that it is an accurate reflection of practices and outcomes.

Medical records

Patients' medical notes are a frequent source of information for many studies and service evaluations. However, their purpose is to document information relevant to patient care and promote good outcomes. Whilst they are a useful source for some investigations, they may not provide a sufficiently comprehensive, systematic and verifiable source of information for many research questions.

Medical records may be paper or electronic. With the rise in electronic prescribing, electronic medication records are increasingly available as a data source. For hospital inpatients, information may be available on the prescribing, dispensing, administration and monitoring of medicines, as well as records of allergy status. Electronic prescribing systems are often able to run analyses of these records for audit, service evaluation and quality improvement purposes at an individual, ward or organisational level. These analyses depend on the correct classification and coding of the information having been inputted and therefore have some limitations. However, they are a useful potential resource for those carrying out medicines-related projects in hospitals.

Stages involved in retrospective studies using medical records and databases may include identifying a relevant database in line with the project aims and objectives, appraising the completeness, reliability and validity of the data, and data extraction. As part of this process it is important to ascertain how the primary data was collected. A data extraction form should also be developed that allows the relevant data to be recorded. Data should be recorded anonymously wherever possible.

The literature as a secondary data source: meta-analysis and data synthesis

Meta-analysis is a process in which data from a number of previous studies are combined into a new dataset. Relevant studies may be drawn from the published literature and, when they can be located, unpublished sources. The larger dataset confers greater statistical power in the application of analytical procedures leading to more reliable results. It is a technique that is applied to tightly structured quantitative studies, especially clinical trials. However, meta-analysis presents many challenges. Studies will vary hugely in their methodology and quality. Variation in the completeness and detail of reporting may make it difficult to be assured of the actual operation and procedures. Research aims, population groups, eligibility criteria, data collection methods and outcome measures may lead to concerns over the comparability of the studies. However, when studies of comparable focus, methodology and sufficient quality can be identified, meta-analysis can be an effective and efficient way of reaching more dependable conclusions regarding a research question.

When a formal statistical analysis cannot be undertaken because of difficulties in ascertaining the quality of studies or the lack of comparability, a *narrative synthesis* may be used to combine findings descriptively. Again, clear eligibility criteria about focus and quality should be applied in the selection of papers. The employment of an appropriate conceptual or theoretical framework may be valuable in facilitating a systematic and local reappraisal of the findings of the combined studies. This should be transparent in its application. A robust approach, possibly involving at least two researchers, should be taken to the extraction of data and interpretation of the findings of the different studies to ensure the reliability of procedures, and hence the validity of the work. In addition to highlighting deficiencies and strengths in a current evidence base, these studies can provide new insights into knowledge and understanding.

Another approach to reanalysis of primary studies is a realist synthesis. This will involve a combining the results of different studies in order to determine which interventions may work for different people in different contexts.

Similar approaches and many of the techniques discussed above can also be applied to combining and synthesis of data and/or findings from different types of study, including qualitative research. Whatever the nature of the studies, principles of scientific enquiry and sound research methodology are paramount if the results of the work are to be of value.

Studies drawing on existing data sources are usually less resource consuming as the time and costs of data collection are avoided. Opportunity costs and competing priorities for research funds may encourage greater exploitation of existing sources of data. Meta-analysis, narrative review and realist reviews can be immensely valuable in making evidence-based recommendation, as well as highlighting the strengths and weaknesses of an evidence base, and identifying priorities for further research.

More information on the different stages in carrying out literature reviews is given in **Chapter 8**.

Documents and other sources

A wide range of written sources may be available to researchers. These may include policy documents or other written material from organisations including government, professional and regulatory bodies, non-government organisations, industry, etc. Information may relate to health policy, professional practice, or needs of specified populations or user groups, down to information designed for individual patients. Sources may be written documents, meeting minutes, reports, newsletters, internet sites, advertisements, leaflets and medicine package inserts, etc. Both qualitative and structured quantitative analytical procedures may be applied. Similar approaches to those employed in the reappraisal of previous research, as discussed above, may be appropriate.

In the analysis of documentary and written sources, both structured quantitative and/or qualitative procedures may be applied. A common structured approach is *content analysis* . This may be applied to describe the content of, for example, information with medicines, advertisements, contents of selected websites, etc. It is often viewed as a quantitative approach that enables the description of the content of sources: frequency with which issues are raised, level of detail provided, presence of different viewpoints, etc. Sometimes content analysis is used to compare similar information from different sources. This structured quantitative approach may be followed by a more *interpretative* one, or an interpretative qualitative approach may be used solely. For example, this may involve the application of phenomenological techniques to examine explicit or implicit goals, values, views or rationales of authors or bodies producing the documents.

Analysis of documents may also be guided by a theoretical or empirical framework, which may combine elements of a structured content analysis with interpretation of meanings and messages.

Research using documentary sources should also be systematic. This applies to the identification and selection of material, as well as the analytical procedures. If the findings are to be generalised, all possible sources of relevant information should be identified, and material selected that is representative. Data processing, coding and analytical procedures should be clear and consistently applied.

Conclusion

Where data exist, which can answer your research question or provide valuable insights into your area of interest, it is sensible to use them. Analysis of databases and secondary analysis can be applied to answer many topical research questions. They can also have an important role in furthering scientific knowledge and understanding and evaluating and informing the operation of organisations, professional practice and patient care.

Analyses of these data still require a high level of scientific enquiry and the application of sound methodological procedures. If you are not embarking on fieldwork and data collection yourself, you still need to have an appreciation of the potential problems that may arise in obtaining high-quality, comprehensive and dependable data. You need to apply critical thought to how you are using the data that you have with regard to its potential reliability and validity for your project. The varied sources of existing data and secondary analyses are increasingly viewed as an important resource for researchers.

Questions

1. Identify five potential sources of primary data.

2. Describe two advantages in carrying out analyses of existing data.

3. Discuss three potential challenges when reanalysing primary data, and how these may be mitigated.

4. Identify three methods of synthesising findings from primary studies.

5. Which one of the following is true of a narrative synthesis?
   A: It can only include qualitative data
   B: It uses statistical analysis to combine findings of different studies
   C: It can be used to synthesise heterogeneous studies

CHAPTER 15

Data processing and analysis

LEARNING OBJECTIVES

Upon completion of this chapter you should be able to:

- understand the principles of, and key procedures for carrying out descriptive quantitative analysis
- select appropriate statistical tests to analyse quantitative data
- understand the principles of, and key procedure for carrying out qualitative data analysis using deductive and inductive approaches
- employ procedures to ensure reliability and validity of analysis.

Data collection is followed by data processing and analysis. Data processing comprises those activities required to prepare the data for analysis. Although many tasks will be common to most studies, these activities will depend to some extent on the type of data and the analytical techniques employed; in particular, distinct approaches are associated with quantitative and qualitative research. The stages of analysis are shown in *Box 15.1*.

Box 15.1: Stages of analysis in primary research

- Collate the data (collect together all questionnaires, interview transcripts, data collection forms, etc.)
- Organise, annotate and/or transcribe data according to the types of study and data, to prepare for subsequent analysis
- Develop a coding frame
- Code all data according to the coding frame
- Enter all coded data into a spreadsheet or a software package for analysis (if this is to be used)
- Do the analysis (as required by the study objectives)

Quantitative research

Quantitative studies are those for which the researcher wishes to count or measure particular phenomena; for example, you may want to count the number of respondents who have had a particular experience or have certain views or attitudes. You may want to establish the frequency of events, the extent to which certain groups of individuals experience problems, or the proportion of patients who are prescribed a particular drug. All these studies will require some counting and quantification of data. It is worth noting that, if you have done a survey of people's views and attitudes to establish the *number* or *proportion* of individuals who hold certain viewpoints, then in your data processing and analysis you will require *quantitative* procedures, despite the apparent subjective nature of your topic.

In quantitative studies, researchers may also wish to examine and quantify relationships between variables; for example, examine associations between the characteristics of respondents or the views, or they may wish to examine whether certain groups of individuals are more likely to act in particular ways or take part in certain events.

Some studies are designed to test a hypothesis. These will involve the application of probability statistics to examine the differences between groups and establish the likelihood that any differences result from real differences between the groups rather than differences that might be expected to occur just by chance.

Quantitative studies (e.g. survey research) often generate large datasets as a result of the number of variables (questions) and/or cases (respondents). In general, questionnaires, structured interviews (i.e. in which a questionnaire is employed in an interview setting), non-participant observation (which often involves the gathering of structured data), prospective recording of events and analysis of existing datasets are methods to which quantitative analytical procedures are applied.

Data processing in quantitative research

Coding frames and coding

The first stage in the processing of quantitative data is the collation of all questionnaires and/or data collection instruments for coding. Before you can code your data, you need to develop a coding frame. The coding frame consists of specification of codes for all variables (e.g. questions in a questionnaire) and all values of (i.e. potential responses to) these variables in the dataset.

As questionnaires generally include a high proportion of closed questions (in which a limited number of response options are provided in the questionnaire), much of the instrument can be precoded, i.e. codes can be decided in advance, and the question laid out so that the respondents indicate their response by circling the appropriate code (*Box 15.2*).

Open questions require an additional stage in data processing. To these questions the respondents can answer in any way that they wish. The coding frame is then usually based on the actual responses made and will often be developed after the data have been collected. For a sample of the questionnaires, the researcher will list the different responses that have been given, attempt to group them together and then assign codes.

Similar procedures will be followed for other standardised data collection instruments, e.g. records of observations, diary entries, data extracted from patient notes, etc.

Missing data must also be coded. When you come to do the analysis, it is important to know about missing data. Data can be 'missing' for different reasons; for example, if a researcher forgot to ask a question, or the respondent did not know the answer or was unwilling to reply. In some cases, a response may be missing for a legitimate reason, e.g. because the question was 'not applicable' to a particular person or case. If a person drops out of a study, or completes only half a questionnaire, there will be consequent missing data.

Different codes should be allocated to data that are missing for different reasons. If a question was 'not applicable' to a number of individuals or cases, then these should be identifiable and omitted from the analysis. If data are missing because respondents chose not to respond or for a reason that is unclear, this could indicate potential problems with the reliability of the data. When analysing the data, it is possible to include or exclude missing, and/or not applicable, cases as appropriate. It is, of course, important to be able to state the number of cases for which data are missing.

Box 15.2: Variables and values: example of questions and coding frame

Questionnaire		Coding frame	
		Sex	
Are you:	Male? □	Male	...1
	Female? □	Female	...2
		Missing	...9
How old were you last birthday?		Age	
		Insert age	____
		Missing	999
Do you currently take any medicines?		Medicines	
Yes	...□	Yes	...1
No	...□	No	...2
If yes,			
How many different products are you currently taking?		Numbered	
		Insert number	____
		Not applicable	98
		Missing	99
How would you describe you health?		Self perceived health	
Excellent	...□	Excellent	...1
Good	...□	Good	...2
Fair	...□	Fair	...3
Poor	...□	Poor	...4
		Missing	...9

A unique code or case number should also be assigned to each respondent (or case) to enable identification. Codes may also be included for contextual information, situational variables or details of the data collection process. For example, if a number of interviewers were involved in the data collection, you could give a code to each and include this as a variable when you code the data. If data were collected in a number of different locations, you may wish to assign a code for each. This would enable you to identify and compare data collected by different individuals or in different places. Codes may also be applied to indicate the date of receipt of a returned questionnaire and/or whether it followed the initial or a subsequent mailing. These factors can then be examined in the analysis.

Coding can be more complicated for questions that allow the respondent to select more than one response (i.e. multiple response items). In the questionnaire, the directions should be clear about how many responses may be selected and whether these should be ranked. For these questions, the coding frame must be designed so that the required analyses can be performed. For some analyses, it may be necessary to code each possible response as if it were a separate variable (question).

The coding frame should also include directions for the researchers with regard to the coding procedures, especially how to code ambiguous or unusual responses, e.g. a decision has to be made by the researchers about how a response should be coded if the respondent ticked two boxes when they were instructed to tick only one. The researchers have to use their judgement in making these decisions; what is important is that these decisions are documented and consistently applied.

Coding the data

Once the coding frame is complete, the data are coded in accordance with the coding frame. The codes will often be entered directly on to each questionnaire or data collection form. The reliability of coding should be checked, especially for open questions that can be difficult to interpret and categorise; detailed instructions in the coding frame are very helpful here. The reliability of the coding procedure can be checked by having a sample of the questionnaires, interview schedules or data collection forms coded by two researchers independently. The codes assigned by the two researchers can then be compared. This is referred to as a check on *inter-rater reliability*.

Data entry

Coded data are entered into a database for analysis. A number of statistical packages are available for this. If only very basic procedures are required, Excel can be used. However, probably the most commonly used is the Statistical Package for the Social Sciences (SPSS). This program allows a wide range of simple and complex statistical procedures that are appropriate for pharmacy practice and related research. Some databases are limited in the analytical procedures that are possible or else are designed for particular purposes. It is important to know what procedures will be needed and to check that the software has the capacity to meet them.

Data entry is a mechanical task, but it is important. Care with data entry and systematic checking is vital. A great deal of work will often have gone into the planning of the study and the data collection. The value of the study can be undermined if data entry is poor. The validity of the analysis depends on how accurately the data are entered; care in avoiding errors can save much work later on. The correction of a single entry can result in having to repeat whole sets of analyses. Conversely, if the coding and data entry procedures are carried out with care and appropriate checking, the analysis should be smooth and often quite speedy.

The process of checking for, identifying and rectifying inaccuracies is referred to as 'cleaning' the data. Cleaning the data may involve a proactive approach including checking the data entered against the original coded instruments and/or conducting frequency analyses on different variables to identify any outliers or spurious entries.

Approaching the analysis

You need a plan for your analysis (*Box 15.3*). This will be guided by the objectives of the study. In terms of the statistical procedures, it should start with straightforward approaches that enable you to understand the characteristics of your dataset before you embark on investigations of associations between variables (bivariate tests) or any more complex procedures.

Box 15.3: A plan for the analysis

- Descriptive procedures: frequencies on each variable, e.g. tables, bar charts, pie charts to provide an overview of the data. Decide for each variable if summary statistics, e.g. mean, median, or a measure of spread – standard deviation, range – would also be informative. This will provide information on the characteristics of respondents or cases: number of males and females, number (and average number) of events, proportion of respondents who report a particular viewpoint or experience, etc.
- Bivariate procedures to examine associations between variables or differences between groups: e.g. cross-tabulations, chi-square tests, Mann–Whitney U (non-parametric data); *t*-tests (normally distributed data).
- Other, perhaps more complex, methods as required by the study objectives.

Software packages for statistical analysis of quantitative (e.g. survey) data are very powerful. They offer the possibility of a great variety of procedures and manipulation of data, many of which will be inappropriate for your data or project.

It is important that when you are approaching and planning the analysis you think about the limitations of the data. Non-random sampling procedures, small datasets, poorly constructed questions, unreliable responses, missing values, etc., all limit the validity of the data. It is important to be realistic about the quality of the data. In survey research it is well recognised that some questions may be problematic, thus affecting the validity of the responses. If, during the data collection or data processing, it becomes apparent that some questions presented difficulties, consideration should be given to the exclusion of these from the analysis.

A further danger arises in that if you perform a large number of tests of relationships between variables, you will inevitably chance upon some statistically significant associations. For example, if a 0.05 level of statistical significance is selected, as is conventional, this means that a relationship between variables is assumed to be real if there is a 95% probability that it would not have occurred by chance, i.e. there is a 1 in 20 chance that the association is spurious. In other words, for every 20 tests performed, one statistically significant result would be expected even if there were no systematic relationships between variables in the dataset. Data analysis in which researchers test for associations between variables in the dataset until they find them are sometimes referred to as 'fishing expeditions'. To avoid the possibility of misleading findings, statisticians advise that the analysis should be planned in advance according to the specific study objectives and that you should stick to this plan.

Software packages for statistical analysis place a huge range of complex and powerful procedures at the disposal of the researcher. Many are simple to perform in that programs are often menu driven. However, this simplicity can mask the complexity of the procedures, most of which rest on complicated assumptions about the structure of the dataset. If these assumptions do not apply, the procedures may be invalid and meaningless. Ensuring that the data conform to the necessary assumptions requires considerable understanding and expertise. Failure to check that these assumptions are not violated can result in a real danger of performing inappropriate analyses, leading to incorrect conclusions.

Selection of statistical procedures for descriptive studies

In the selection of the appropriate analytical procedures, the characteristics of the data in terms of, first, the type of variable and, second, the distribution of the values as parametric (usually normally distributed) or non-parametric (distribution-free) must be determined. These are often straightforward to ascertain and enable you to select appropriate procedures.

Types of variable

In quantitative research, data relating to each variable may be (*Box 15.4*):

- nominal: in which a value or code is assigned to each of the possible responses which have no inherent order or ranking, e.g. male = 1, female = 2; or yes = 1, no = 2
- ordinal: where codes are applied, and the value of the code represents increasing value of the variable, e.g. occasionally = 1, sometimes = 2, often = 3
- interval/ratio: where the value or code represents a true value, e.g. total serum cholesterol or the number of prescription medicines currently prescribed for an individual. For interval data, the distance between the points on the scale will be proportionate.

Box 15.4: Examples of categorical, ordinal and interval/ratio data

Categorical data:
Male = 1
Female = 2
Respondent reports reading information leaflet = 1
Respondent does not read information leaflet = 2

Ordinal data:
How would you describe your health?

Excellent	1
Good	2
Fair	3
Poor	4

How satisfied are you with your pharmacy services?

Always	1
Mostly	2
Sometimes	3
Occasionally	4
Never	5

Interval data:
How many medicines are you currently prescribed?
Clinical measures, e.g. blood pressure, BMI, HbA1c

Parametric and non-parametric data

Many statistical tests depend on the data conforming to known probability distribution. When this is the case, statistical procedures which are based on normal distribution theory can be employed. In other situations, non-parametric tests are more appropriate; in general these are less powerful.

Parametric data

Probability statistics used in research are commonly based on the normal distribution and interval data. In the application of these techniques there is an underlying assumption that the data are normally distributed. Data that are normally distributed, when plotted out, fall into a 'bell-shaped' distribution. The mean (middle) value is at the apex of the curve, which is symmetrical (similar numbers of cases above and below the mean, and a similar spread of cases either side of the mean). The standard deviation is a measure of the distance from the mean (above and below) that includes 68% of cases, thus it is a measure of how close to or how far from the mean most of the cases lie.

Non-parametric data

Many biochemical and physiological measures (e.g. height, weight, blood pressure in a population, etc.) naturally fall into a normal distribution. However, for other variables this may not be so. Commonly, in health service and pharmacy practice research, many variables are not normally distributed and for these, non-parametric (distribution-free) procedures, which do not depend on the data being distributed in any particular way, should be applied. For example, the number of prescription drugs regularly taken by a population would not be expected to be normally distributed (a high proportion of the population may take none or one, and progressively fewer take larger numbers). Journey times to a pharmacy may also be skewed, with most of the population living within a very short distance away, whereas small numbers have very long journey times. If data are not normally distributed, or when the dependent variable being tested is ordinal rather than interval, non-parametric analytical procedures should be employed (*Box 15.5*).

Box 15.5: Normally and non-parametrically distributed variables

Variables likely to be normally distributed:
- Clinical measures, e.g. blood pressure, BMI (body mass index), HbA1c (glycated haemoglobin)

Variables that are less likely to be normally distributed (these distributions are likely to be skewed to the left):
- Number of prescribed medicines
- Number of medicine-related problems
- Waiting times in a pharmacy

Planning your analysis

Descriptive procedures and summary statistics are often the first stage in the analysis of data in any research project (*Box 15.6*).

Box 15.6: Procedures that are commonly employed in quantitative studies

- Frequency analyses: tables, bar charts, pie charts to display the characteristics of the variables in a dataset. These can be applied to all variables whether nominal, ordinal or interval/ratio.
- Summary statistics: middle values: mean (normally distributed interval data), median (an alternative to the mean for data that are not normally distributed). Measures of spread of the data include, for normally distributed data, the standard deviation, which indicates the distance from the mean of the majority (68%) of cases. For non-parametric data, the range (maximum and minimum values) or interquartile ranges may be reported.
- Investigations of associations between the variables in the dataset, e.g. cross-tabulations, chi-square tests, *t*-tests, Wilcoxon's signed ranks tests and Mann–Whitney U tests, correlation (Spearman's rank and least squares).
- More complex investigations of association between variables can be performed using multivariate methods (procedures that are performed on data relating to three or more variables simultaneously). These procedures include regression, analysis of variance, factor analysis, some modelling procedures, etc.

Often the first stage of analysis in a descriptive study is to obtain frequency data on most, or all, of the variables in the dataset. This provides descriptive information on all respondents according to their responses to the questions, e.g. the number of male and female respondents, their age group, work location, views on particular issues, number of prescription-related problems recorded, etc., according to the questionnaire.

This information can be supplemented by summary statistics. Rather than list all the values, reporting the mean or median values or a measure of the spread of the values may be helpful. If data are normally distributed, the mean value (arithmetic average = sum of all values/number of cases) can be reported. In normally distributed data the mean and the median will be similar. The median (middle value) is used in non-parametric data. This provides an indication of the value that is characteristic of an 'average' member of the population. In datasets in which a small proportion of the population report unusually high values, this will be reflected in a higher population mean. The median value may then be a more useful reflection of a typical population value for a variable that is skewed by the presence of a small number of unusually low or high values, i.e. outliers.

Measures of spread of data include standard deviation (for normally distributed data), maximum and minimum values, and interquartile ranges. If the data are normally distributed, the standard deviation is very informative because two-thirds of cases will lie within one standard deviation of the mean and 95% will lie within two standard deviations.

Investigating associations between categorical variables

If the dataset is sufficiently large, associations between different variables in a dataset can be investigated, e.g. between age of respondent and number of prescribed medicines, or location of pharmacy and workload. Selection of the best procedure is governed by the type of data (as nominal, ordinal or interval/ratio) and the distribution of the values (as normal or non-normal).

Test of difference between groups

Nominal data (categorical data)
Cross-tabulation of data enables documentation of the number of cases according to predetermined categories. A table is constructed that categorises each case according to the response to each of two variables, thus forming a cell structure (*Table 15.1*). A chi-square test may then be performed to indicate whether the number of cases in each cell departs from that which would be expected if there were no association between the variables. For example, to investigate whether male or female pharmacists were more or less likely to respond to a questionnaire, a chi-square test would compare the actual number of male and female respondents and non-respondents with the numbers that would be expected if there were no systematic differences between them. From the chi-square statistic, the probability that the responses represent a systematic difference between the groups can be ascertained.

For the chi-square test to be valid there should be an expected frequency of at least five cases in each cell. Also, a correction factor is required for small (2×2 tables, i.e. one degree of freedom) tables. Care is required with large tables (i.e. variables for which there are a large number of categories/values) as the test itself does not specify where any differences lie.

Table 15.1: *Example of cross-tabulation and chi-square test*

	Responded to questionnaire	Did not respond	Total
Males	81 (expected: 120 × 146/230 = 76)	39 (expected: 44)	120
Females	65 (expected: 70)	45 (expected: 40)	110
Total	146	84	230

Chi-square = 1.53, degree of freedom (df) = 1

Reference to tables indicates that a chi-square value of 1.53 (with 1 df) is below the threshold of 3.84, which would indicate statistical significance at the 5% level (i.e. $p < 0.05$). Thus, we would conclude that there is no systematic difference in the response rates between male and female participants.

If the expected frequency is less than five cases in each cell, a Fisher's exact test can be performed instead.

Ordinal data and non-normally distributed interval data
Non-parametric procedures are used to investigate the possible statistical significance of differences between groups when data are either ordinal or do not form a normal distribution. To compare data from two groups (e.g. male and female respondents) a Wilcoxon signed rank test (for paired data, i.e. the same group of respondent is tested at more than one point in time) or the Mann–Whitney U test (for unpaired data, i.e. where two different group of respondents are compared) is commonly performed (*Box 15.7*). This is based on rankings of all cases according to the variable of interest. The ranks for the two groups are then compared and assessed to establish the likelihood that the differences in the ranks could have occurred by chance. The Kruskal–Wallis test is a similar procedure employed when more than two groups are being compared.

Box 15.7: Application of a Mann–Whitney U test

A Mann–Whitney U test was carried out to establish if prescribers who had attended a training programme were more likely to adhere to guidelines in the prescribing practice than those who had not attended.

Adherence to prescribing guidelines was measured using an (ordinal) scale (assessing choice of formulation, dose, duration of therapy) on which each prescriber achieved a score. The scores were not normally distributed, so a non-parametric rather than a *t*-test was required.

A Mann–Whitney U test was performed to compare the scores of the two groups. A *p* value = 0.023 was obtained, with prescribers who had attended the course achieving higher scores (greater adherence with guidelines) than those who had not.

Thus, it was concluded that prescribers who had attended the course were significantly more likely ($p < 0.05$) to adhere to prescribing guidelines.

Interval/ratio data that are normally distributed

To compare two groups of respondents on a normally distributed variable, a paired or unpaired *t*-test can be performed (*Box 15.8*). This compares the mean values for each group and, based on normal distribution theory, assesses whether the difference is likely to have occurred by chance or to represent a real difference between the two groups. Analysis of variance (ANOVA) can be used to assess differences between more than two groups.

Box 15.8: A *t*-test

The number of hours of study per week undertaken by first and final year pharmacy students was compared. A sample of students from each cohort kept diaries in which they recorded their hours of study. Analysis of data revealed that first years studied on average 37 hours/week. The standard deviation (SD) of 6 hours indicated that 95% of students studied between 31 and 43 hours. For final year students the mean was 43 hours (SD = 6.2).

Data conformed adequately to a normal distribution. Thus, a *t*-test was performed, which confirmed that differences in study hours between the two groups was statistically significant ($p < 0.05$). It was therefore concluded that there were real differences between first and final year students in their study habits.

Associations between two ordered or continuous variables (tests of correlation)

Correlation is used to assess the relationship between two ordered or continuous variables, i.e. the extent to which an increase in one variable is associated with an increase in the other (e.g. the extent to which blood pressure rises with age) (*Box 15.9*). Non-parametric procedures (e.g. Spearman's rank correlation) are used for ordinal or non-normally distributed data. Simple linear correlation (e.g. Pearson's correlation) can be used for normally distributed data. Before the calculation of a correlation coefficient, a scatter plot should be drawn to assess the appropriateness of the procedure, e.g. there may be a relationship between the values of the variables that is not linear and would not be identified by this procedure.

Box 15.9: Correlation between variables

Providing assistance with medicines can be burdensome and stressful for many family members or carers. An interview study was undertaken in which data on levels of carer stress (measured on an established ordinal scale) and the number of medicines-related problems experienced by carers (interval data) were collected.

The variables did not fall into a normal distribution, but a scatter plot showed that there was a roughly linear relationship between them. Spearman's rank correlation was performed.

This revealed a statistically significant relationship (correlation coefficient 0.34; $p < 0.001$) between levels of stress and number of medicines-related problems, i.e. as the number of medicines-related problems increased, so did levels of stress experienced by carers.

Multivariate procedures

The procedures outlined above involve the analysis of data relating to two variables at a time. These bivariate procedures are commonly employed in the initial investigations of relationships between variables. Procedures that analyse data relating to three or more variables simultaneously are referred to as multivariate. Multivariate procedures assume that the variables will be interrelated, i.e. that a change in the value of one variable will be accompanied by a change in the value of others. In these circumstances it is seen as appropriate to adopt a multivariate approach to the analysis. Computer software provides opportunities for researchers to undertake complex and exciting procedures in the analysis of their data. The common packages designed for the analysis of quantitative (especially survey) data offer a wide range of multivariate procedures.

It is beyond the scope of this text to detail the wide range of multivariate procedures that may be performed. However, by way of an overview, multivariate procedures are sometimes classified as dependence methods, in which one or more variables are identified as the variables of interest (dependent variable(s)). Analytical procedures then focus on explaining changes in the values of the dependent variables in terms of others, i.e. independent variables. Examples of these procedures are multiple regression, discriminant analysis and multivariate analysis of variance (MANOVA).

Regression is one of the most common, more complex procedures used in the analysis of quantitative data. This is a technique to identify variables (independent variables) that are predictive of a variable of interest (dependent variable), e.g. to identify factors that are predictive of the level of consumption of non-prescription medicines. Logistic regression is employed when the dependent variable takes on two nominal values. Discriminant analysis may provide an alternative to logistic regression. In this procedure, independent variables are combined into a new variable that distinguishes between individuals in terms of the dependent variable. MANOVA is similar to ANOVA in that it assesses differences between groups, but on the basis of more than one dependent variable.

Other procedures are classified as interdependence methods. These are where the variables are analysed as a single interrelated set, none of which is designated as dependent or otherwise of particular importance for the purposes of the analysis. Factor and cluster analyses are examples of these procedures.

Factor analysis has been widely used in survey work in pharmacy practice, especially in studies of people's beliefs and attitudes. It is a data reduction technique that is used to reduce a larger number of variables to a smaller number of underlying dimensions or factors. Cluster analysis enables individuals or cases to be distinguished or grouped (into clusters) in terms of other variables in the dataset.

Multivariate analyses are complicated. A limited understanding of the underlying mathematics and assumptions of these procedures risks their inappropriate use. Their availability in common software packages for the analysis of survey data can lead to their application to datasets that were not designed with these procedures in mind. Great care must be taken to ensure the validity of their application. If they are to be used, it may be helpful if a statistician is also involved.

Inferential statistics

Much research is based on data derived from a sample rather than the whole population. Confidence intervals enable the extrapolation of findings, based on the sample estimates, to the population from which the sample was drawn (assuming that a probability sampling procedure was followed). The calculation of confidence intervals is based on normal distribution theory. Thus, for normally distributed data, the width of the confidence intervals provides an indication of how accurate the estimate (derived from the sample) is likely to be when applied to the study population. A confidence interval (conventionally 95%) consists of two values; one of which will be below and the other above the sample mean. Thus, although not able to state the precise population mean value, the researcher can be 95% sure that it is between these two values.

Measurement scales

Likert scales: Instruments to investigate people's views and beliefs commonly comprise a series of questions or items to which participants respond on a Likert scale (strongly agree, agree, neither agree nor disagree, disagree, strongly disagree). Frequency analysis will usually be the first stage of the analysis of the data. This will be a report of the number or percentage of respondents who strongly agree, agree, neither agree nor disagree, disagree or strongly disagree with each statement. These results may also be presented as bar charts.

As a result of the non-linearity of the Likert scale, the validity of assigning numeric values of 1-5 to responses to the items is questionable. A response of disagree and strongly disagree may reflect similar viewpoints or experiences, but a neutral response or agreement may signify a very different line of thought. Similarly, the validity of summing scores across different items or questions must also be carefully considered. Factor analysis is sometimes used to identify components of these beliefs or views. Cronbach's alpha is a measure of reliability that is commonly applied to assess the internal consistency of the items of a scale. This measure is based on the intra-correlations between the different items of a scale that are believed to be measuring the same attribute or dimension.

By contrast, assumptions of linearity are made in respect of visual analogue scales. It is assumed that when presented with an unanchored visual analogue scale the respondent 'visualises' the line as representing a single dimension when formulating their response.

Scales are also used in the measurement of health status, quality of life, adherence to medicines and many other phenomena. Many of these will have been validated and will have set procedures that must be followed when the data are analysed. It is important that these instructions are followed.

Statistical analysis in intervention studies

As with descriptive studies, the first step in the analysis may be to present frequency data to enable examination of the important characteristics of, and differences between, the datasets. However, in analysing the data from intervention or experimental studies, additional procedures are employed that focus on testing for statistically significant differences between the groups (intervention and control).

It would be unlikely in any study for the results from two groups to be identical even if an intervention had had no impact. Statistical procedures are used to assess whether the differences between the intervention and control groups represent real differences between the two datasets or whether they probably just occurred by chance. Thus, tests of statistical significance are conducted.

A statistical significance test is based on the assumption that the two datasets (intervention and control) could have come from the 'same population', or that there is no evidence of a real difference between the two groups. This is sometimes referred to as the 'null hypothesis'. Two samples from the same population may not be identical, but they should be similar. The question that is asked is: based on the similarities (or differences) between the two sets of data (intervention and control group), what is the chance that both come from the same population (or that there is no real difference between them)? If, based on probability statistics, the differences between the two samples suggest that it is likely that there are no real differences between them are such that the chances are that they are from the same population is very small, we may decide to accept that there is a real difference between the two groups. By convention, in much research p values of less than 0.05 (or 5%) are often taken as conferring statistical significance, i.e. there is a less than 5% probability that the differences between the two groups would have occurred by chance.

When reporting the results, it is usual to report summary statistics for each of the groups on all the relevant variables. This will indicate the size of differences between the intervention and control groups, as well as establishing whether or not the difference is statistically significant.

Qualitative research

Data processing and analysis in qualitative research employ a very different range of techniques from quantitative research. Small numbers of respondents, but often large amounts of textual data, are a feature of the datasets of these studies. Data are commonly verbatim transcripts of semi-structured or in-depth interviews and transcripts of discussions of focus groups. Qualitative approaches are also employed in the analysis of detailed field notes of observations by researchers and case studies. Analysis of qualitative data is a highly skilled task. There are numerous texts dedicated to the description and rationale of possible approaches and procedures.

Approaches to data processing and analysis

The approach to data processing and analysis will depend on the study objectives, in particular the extent to which the researcher follows purist principles of qualitative enquiry (e.g. unstructured interviews), as opposed to a more structured framework determined by their preset objectives or agenda. Thus, the goals of the research may range from the development of theories or hypotheses to explain phenomena of interest, to the provision of detailed descriptions of respondents' views or experiences with regard to specific situations or events. These goals will influence the approach to data collection, processing and analysis.

All qualitative studies require observance of principles of qualitative enquiry such that the data are a true and comprehensive reflection of the perspective of the respondents. Just as when collecting the data, the researchers have to ensure that their procedures and techniques are sensitive to respondents' views and thoughts. The data processing and analysis are also constructed to enable a full and accurate representation of these perspectives.

Grounded theory and framework approaches

Grounded theory or framework approaches are the most commonly employed techniques in the analysis of qualitative data. Grounded theory is theory generated from empirical research. It is often considered a more purist approach to qualitative enquiry. The researcher maintains an open mind and allows themes, ideas and explanations of phenomena to emerge from the data, rather than applying a predetermined framework to the analysis of data. This *inductive* approach is a central feature of grounded theory. Emergent themes, descriptions, explanations of phenomena, etc., are then examined in the context of the natural settings and situations in which they occur. A process of *constant comparison* (see further) is often employed. Through repeated data collection, processing and analysis, theory is developed, refined and verified.

For many studies in health services research, including some into aspects of medicines use and professional practice, a pure grounded theory approach may not be appropriate. In health services and other applied research, researchers may have specific goals and a *priori* research questions which provide a framework for both data collection (often semi-structured instruments) and analysis. However, a qualitative approach will enable an examination of issues of interest in a holistic manner, in the context of natural settings and from the perspective of the people under study. The analysis of data may draw on *deductive* and *inductive* techniques. A deductive approach draws on preidentified theories, ideas or priorities that provide a framework (often the initial basis for the coding structure) to guide the analysis. However, within this framework, the researcher will endeavour to employ an inductive approach applying techniques of constant comparison.

Procedures of data processing and analysis (*Box 15.10*)

The first stage in the data processing of qualitative material is generally verbatim transcription of interviews. This can be a very time-consuming task. One 20-minute interview will usually take several hours to transcribe. A lengthy focus group discussion may take several days. Contextual data from field notes may also be included. When planning your study, you should make sure that you build in enough time for transcription of data. Analysis of large quantities of transcribed data can also be extremely time-consuming if it is to be done well.

Box 15.10: Stages in qualitative data processing and analysis

- Transcription of data:
  - and familiarisation with issues
  - entry into computer software package to facilitate data handling (optional)
- Development of a primary coding frame:
  - based on content of transcripts, i.e. perspectives of respondents regarding the relevant issues according to and/or informed by study objectives
  - Coding of data: application of codes to the data (sometimes referred to as indexing)
- Development of more detailed coding frames:
  - to allow a more questioning examination of issues and phenomena
  - to identify participants' perspectives regarding possible explanations for phenomena and/or their rationale for behaviours or beliefs
  - to distinguish specific contextual or situational factors that may be pertinent to the interpretation of the data
  - to enable cross-linking between issues relevant to more than one principal theme
- Examination of issues both within cases and between cases
- Checks on the validity and reliability: active employment of specific techniques to support claims regarding the reliability of procedures and the validity of the study findings

---

Devising a coding frame is commonly the next step after the transcription of data. In qualitative research, whether principles of a grounded approach or framework analysis are to be followed, the structure and content of the coding frame will be derived from, or informed by, the data themselves, i.e. it is devised so that it reflects the issues, descriptions, explanations, etc., provided by respondents. Thus, unlike some quantitative studies, in which coding frames can be developed at the same time as the instrument, and questionnaires sometimes precoded, in qualitative work development of the coding frame has to follow data collection.

The first step in the development of a coding frame is for the researchers to familiarise themselves with the data; this will be achieved to a large extent during the process of transcription. Researchers will then commonly aim to identify a thematic framework that covers all the issues raised by the respondents. Identification of principal themes from within the dataset and their organisation into a framework (which may be just a list of distinct topic areas) may form the primary coding structure.

These primary codes can then be applied to the dataset to enable identification of all data relevant to each of these themes or topic areas within the dataset, i.e. sections of the data that relate to each of these themes are identified and codes are inserted. The application of codes to the data is sometimes referred to as *indexing*. During the application of these primary codes to the data, some additional themes or topics may emerge, necessitating some revision of the primary coding frame. These may be the identification of new issues (that do not fit existing codes), which therefore require new codes, or the subdivision of some themes into distinct topic areas requiring additional codes.

After identification of the principal themes, the researcher may then embark on a more detailed examination of data within each of these areas. This may involve the development of a separate coding structure for data relating to each of the principal themes. Themes may be subdivided, with different codes used to distinguish specific situational factors or types of explanation provided by the respondents. The researcher may also wish to build into the coding structure the capacity to cross-link issues, situational factors, explanations, etc., relevant to more than one principal theme. In qualitative work, data processing and analysis are likely to be integrated and iterative. New categories or codes and/or subdivisions of existing categories may arise throughout. A coding frame is exhaustive and represents all data items and perspectives.

Constant comparison

The coding frame, to some extent, will evolve as the analysis proceeds. It must enable the organisation of the data so as to facilitate its examination, interpretation and analysis. As the analysis proceeds, new questions or hypotheses may arise that the researcher will want to investigate. There may also be continual formulation and reformulation of hypotheses. This is sometimes referred to as *analytic induction*. It may lead to the development of further levels of coding to enable identification and indexing of all material that may be relevant. A technique of *constant comparison* is often employed. This involves the continual appraisal of items of data by asking the question: 'How does this instance of x differ from previous instances?'. The researcher compares each new item of data with other items to which the same code has been applied, and considers ways in which it is similar to or different from those already coded. For example, differences may relate to context, potential explanatory factors, and or/its meaning from the respondent's point of view. This enables the coding frame and analysis to represent the full diversity of perspectives in the dataset. It helps ensure that hypotheses or theories are continually tested and/or refined. Constant comparison highlights the differences between data items that share the same 'code' so that these differences can inform any theory building process. This contrasts with quantitative analysis in which once items are coded, any contextual or otherwise meaningful differences between cases are no longer the subject of further examination.

Constant comparison maximises the opportunities to provide explanations for phenomena, taking into account the complex situational and other factors that may be important.

Possible questions to ask:

- What is common between cases (A, B and C), and how can similarities be explained?
- What is different between instances (X and Y)? Why?
  And then:
- Do these explanations hold for other instances of M? When? Why/Why not?

Analysis may be performed both within cases, e.g. to examine specific instances of any issue or event in the context of circumstances and other explanatory factors, and between cases to examine apparently similar experiences or events across cases.

Coding and analysis are commonly iterative and interactive. After modifications and refinements to the coding frame, or the development of a new code, the revised coding frame must then be applied systematically to all cases. This can mean recoding all data, and continual appraisal and reappraisal of the dataset and individual items. Qualitative analysis is *interpretative*, continually posing questions to illuminate explanations for, and meanings of, data. It is also a dynamic process; new questions and issues emerging throughout which require modification of procedures and reappraisal of data.

The goal of qualitative analysis is not to present numbers or frequencies of events, views or phenomena. The sampling procedures do not support generalisations to individuals or settings beyond those studied. However, the goal of qualitative research is to examine questions of '*how?*' and '*why?*' particular situations or beliefs emerge, and to explain their impact on behaviours or events. It is assumed that the findings of any qualitative study will be of relevance to other individuals and settings which share particular characteristics and/or where circumstances are similar. Thus, some researchers argue that the use of numbers to provide an indication of the extent to which participants share views and experiences can be helpful in the interpretation of data.

Data management and use of software

Management of the data requires good organisation on the part of the researcher. Datasets can be very large. Although there may be just a small number of interviews/cases, qualitative research can generate large amounts of detailed data, sometimes combining interviews with observation, field notes, and/or documentary sources. Sifting through data by hand to extract the relevant sections can be time-consuming, but in very small studies this may be the most appropriate option. For larger datasets, use of a software package may be preferable. A number of computer packages are available to assist in a comprehensive and systematic approach to coding an analysis. Commonly used software applications include NVivo and MAXQDA. The packages act as repositories for data and, once coded, aid its navigation and retrieval. Through various features including different levels of coding structures, retrieval and display of coded data, facilities for researcher notes/memos, etc., they may also facilitate the analysis of data. For example, to aid a framework approach, data may be summarised into matrices which facilitate thematic and cross-case analysis. Also, some packages can work with data in various different languages.

As these packages are designed to support a systematic approach, they may also be helpful in validation processes. For example, by enabling the efficient identification of all instances in which a topic is raised, they may facilitate a comprehensive approach to argumentative validation (see below).

Reliability and validity in qualitative work

Analysis of qualitative data (as interviewing) is a skilled task. Interpretation by the researcher is an important part of the analytical process. Thus, steps must be taken to ensure the reliability of procedures (*Box 15.11*) and the validity of findings.

Box 15.11: Reliability and validity in qualitative work

Reliability
- Analysis must be systematic and not subjective.
- In development of coding frames there should be agreement between independent researchers.
- In the coding of data there should be agreement between independent researchers:
  - Many responses could fall into more than one category
  - Data are open to interpretation
- All relevant issues and perspectives raised by respondents should be identified and included in the analysis.

Validity
- Are the study findings a 'true' representation of phenomena under study?
- Does the coding frame accurately reflect the true meaning of data?
  - Are there different ways of interpreting and coding the data?
  - In what ways does any conceptual framework influence the interpretation of data?

Reflexivity
- How have the perspectives of the researcher influenced the processes and interpretation of data?
  - Has the researcher taken steps to address the impact of his or her own perspectives and values on the procedures of analysis and interpretation of data?
- In the research process: to what extent are research findings an 'artefact of the methodology'?

Reliability

Two or more researchers may be involved in the development of the coding frame, possibly independently devising their own structures, which are then compared.

As with quantitative work, codes must be consistently applied to the data. As a check on the reliability of the coding process, it is common for this to be undertaken by two researchers independently for a sample of the transcripts. Any discrepancies in the coding must be examined and the coding frame revised to ensure its consistent application.

Validity

In qualitative work it is important that *all* issues and perspectives raised by respondents are included in the analysis. An experience or viewpoint may be raised by only one respondent, and it could be that it is of minor importance. However, on the other hand, it may be explained by particular situational or circumstantial factors, and a pertinent focus of analysis in a qualitative dataset.

The validity of the results (i.e. the extent to which they are a true representation of phenomena under study) must also be assured. There are many opportunities for bias to colour the analytical process. A number of approaches can be employed to validate research findings:

- In the course of the analysis, the researcher may attempt to use the data to argue a viewpoint contradictory to the tentative conclusions or theories, i.e. the researcher will (acting as the devil's advocate) take a systematic approach to looking for examples in the data that do not fit with his or her hypothesis or conclusions.
- After data analysis, the researcher may collect additional data to verify a hypothesis, or ask the original participants to comment on the extent to which they believe that the findings accurately represent their experiences and perspectives. This could be in terms of their description, possible explanations and the complexity.
- Researchers may compare their findings with those of other studies (in the literature) or relevant theory to assess the extent to which they are consistent. Where findings do concur, what does the study add? Where findings do not concur, what further questions are raised?

A systematic and scientific approach to the analysis of qualitative data is of paramount importance to the research. Sound methodological principles and strategies must be rigorously observed if the findings are to be dependable.

Focus groups

In general, the principles of qualitative analysis discussed above apply to focus group data. As for one-to-one interviews, the first stage in the processing of data is verbatim transcriptions of the group discussions, with all contributions correctly assigned to the right participants. Coding frames and coding procedures are then devised as for other qualitative data. However, there are a few additional considerations which are discussed below.

Focus group methodology is often selected because it generally generates a wide-ranging discussion, enabling the identification of many viewpoints. Thus, a common additional goal in the analysis of data is to identify and list the range of perspectives on any issue that are reported by the members of the group. This often includes the extent to which views and experiences of participants differ and/or are similar. This is largely a descriptive process. However, in the analysis researchers will often also want to examine the rationale behind, or reasoning of, participants when explaining their views.

It is the group interaction that provides an added dimension and distinguishes the analytical process from that of one-to-one interviews, and this is often one of the reasons that focus group methodology is selected in the first place. Assuming that all contributions are attributed to the correct participant, the researcher will be able to trace and compare the views, perspectives and experiences of individual participants. They may also be able to investigate if, how and why the views of individuals changed during the course of the discussion.

Group members will usually have been selected because they share some relevant experiences, interests or views. A well-facilitated group discussion between the participants can be very informative in providing insights into service provision, problems, or concerns associated with the aspects of the use of medicines, or professional practices. This is often a goal of the analysis.

Conclusion

The approaches to, and procedures of, data processing and analysis in quantitative and qualitative research differ greatly. However, observance of sound methodological principles and care in maintaining a rigorous approach are essential. Without this, all stages of data processing and analysis are open to practices that may undermine the reliability and validity of the work. A careful and thorough approach (especially in qualitative studies) can be time-consuming; however, it also facilitates a smooth-running analysis, a rewarding path of discovery and findings in which you have confidence.

Questions

1. Which one of these variables is an interval variable?
   A: Number of years since diagnosis
   B: Patient satisfaction with pharmacy services
   C: Gender

Which is the most appropriate statistical test to choose in each of the following circumstances?

2. To test the whether females are more likely to carry records about their medicines than males

3. To test whether patients with mental health conditions are likely to have a higher number of medicine discrepancies when admitted to hospital than those who do not

4. To test whether patients' adherence to medicines is associated with how involved they are during consultations about medicines (both outcome measures being Likert scales)

5. How are inductive and deductive approaches to analysis distinguished?

6. Describe three ways of improving validity in relation to qualitative analysis.

7. Describe two ways of enhancing reliability in relation to qualitative analysis.

CHAPTER 16

Writing the project report/research paper

LEARNING OBJECTIVES

Upon completion of this chapter you should be able to:

- identify the key sections that should be present in a project report and research paper
- identify the information that should be included in each section
- identify appropriate ways of presenting research findings.

After undertaking your project, writing it up is an important part of the research process. Your project report, in addition to fulfilling the requirements for the award of a degree, should be of a quality and standard to enable wider dissemination of the findings. If you have some interesting results that you believe to be valuable, you will want to ensure that these can reach interested audiences and that your achievements can be acknowledged. This chapter focuses on the final project report, providing guidance on its organisation, content and presentation. **Chapter 17** discusses wider dissemination to other audiences and stakeholders.

When to write up

Writing up the report is generally seen as a final stage of any research project. However, it is a good plan not to leave this right until the end. Of course, it is not possible to write up the results or discussion until the work is just about complete, but the introduction and methods can be started at an earlier stage. For most projects the final weeks can be quite pressurised. Inevitably, throughout the study you will have more and less busy times. Typically, at the start of the project you may have to wait for ethical approval or permission from other bodies. During data collection you may be dependent on the availability of others before you can proceed. You should consider this waiting time as valuable, enabling you to undertake the literature review and prepare the introduction to your project.

During those times when the study is under way, but you have to wait for the decisions and cooperation of others, you can commence the writing of your methodology and method. It is a good time to do it when the details about decisions on all aspects of study procedures, preparation of documentation, development of instruments, dealings with ethics committees, liaison with others, etc., are still fresh in your mind. Writing up of the methods section will be greatly aided if you have been making careful notes on your thoughts and decisions about the direction and procedures of the project from the start. You can use these notes to explain why you have done things in certain ways.

Content and organisation of the final report/paper

The project report will usually be very detailed. If the project was undertaken as part of a degree programme, there may be guidelines about the content, presentation, length, style of referencing, etc., of the report. However, it will usually comprise of the following sections:

- Title page
- Acknowledgements
- Summary or abstract
- Introduction with a statement of the aims and objectives
- Methods

- Results
- Discussion
- Conclusion (and recommendations)
- References
- Appendices

Title page

The title page includes the title of the project, the name of the author and their affiliation/position, the institution from which the research was carried out and the date of completion. If the research was conducted as part of the requirement for a degree programme, this is usually also stated.

The acknowledgements

The acknowledgements are an opportunity for the researcher to thank anyone who helped in the research. This may include people who provided guidance or advice on any part of the study, people who helped in identifying and contacting respondents, anyone who assisted in the data collection and, last but not least, the participants themselves. This last group cannot be mentioned by name, because anonymity must be preserved, but they are usually the most important people in any study.

At this point any funding body should be acknowledged. You may also wish to include people who assisted with proofreading or commenting on earlier drafts.

The summary or abstract

This is generally one or two pages in length. Even though it appears at the beginning of the report it is often one of the last sections to be written. It provides an overview of the study and will often include a brief description of the background to the study, objectives, the main methods used, and important findings and conclusions. The abstract is important. It is likely to be the section from which any reviewers obtain their first impressions. Many people will read the abstract first and use it to decide if they want to delve further. A well-written abstract should provoke the reader into reading the rest of the report. It should also be standalone and tell a mini story of the project.

The four main sections

The introduction (with a statement of aims and objectives), methods, results and discussion form the main body of the report. This 'IMRD' structure is the usual way in which empirical scientific research is presented. It tells a story from the background to the topic, explaining why the study was necessary in the first place, what you did and why you did it in particular ways, what you found and what it all means. The aims and objectives are a central part of this. The introduction should set the scene and the research gap; this should directly lead into the aims and objectives. The methods should explain how the objectives will be met. It is often also helpful to structure your results around the objectives. Finally, the extent to which the aims and objectives have been met should be clear in the discussion section. Many journals ask for three points already known about the research area and three points that your paper adds to this knowledge. Whether or not this is required, it may be a useful exercise to undertake to help you structure your story.

The structure and content of each of the four sections invariably require careful thought. The information should be presented in a very straightforward and logical way so that it is easy for the reader to follow. However, all the relevant information must be included. Some general guidance for each of these sections is provided below.

Introduction

The introduction should explain to the reader why the study has been undertaken, i.e. it builds the case for the study. It will usually include a review of the literature identifying other studies relevant to the research area. It should include some critical evaluation of these works, in terms of their strengths and weaknesses (e.g. comments on how a study was done, whether the topic was comprehensively addressed, what questions it left unanswered, or what new issues were raised). Reference should also be made to relevant policy documents or directions in health service provision, professional agendas or practice developments that will demonstrate why the research is important and topical.

The findings from individual papers should be drawn together. After reading the introduction the reader should understand the background to the study and be able to see how the work will add to existing research literature and/or provide important information for specific policy objectives.

The introduction usually leads into a statement of the aims and objectives, or the research question of the project.

Methods

In writing this section attention should be paid to both the methodology and the methods. The section provides an explanation and justification for the methods chosen (i.e. the methodology) and a detailed description of the actual methods used.

For any research topic there may be a number of possible ways of addressing the research questions and obtaining the data required. Each will have its advantages and disadvantages in terms of application of the findings, feasibility, efficiency, costs, reliability, ethical problems, etc. In this section you should explain why particular approaches and methods were chosen and discuss any underlying assumptions and their strengths and weaknesses. This should be done for all stages of the method (sampling strategy, methods of data collection, development of instruments, procedures for validation, etc.).

The methods section must have a logical structure. To achieve this it is often helpful to use subheadings. For example, the methods section may include the following subsections:

- Preliminary fieldwork and piloting
- Ethical and/or local approval, obtaining permission from other bodies
- Inclusion and exclusion criteria
- Sampling strategy and procedures/sources and selection of data
- Recruitment of participants
- Development of the instruments and data collection methods
- Data processing and analysis

It is important to demonstrate to the reader that the methods were robust, acceptable to participants, and well tested. You should attempt to identify and discuss any potential concerns or difficulties in carrying out the study. Preliminary fieldwork that informed decisions about the methodology should be reported. Any revisions to the procedures or instruments as a result of the pilot work should be detailed. When reporting how you selected and recruited your sample, you could also describe the follow up of non-responders, and the steps taken to ensure the reliability of validity of procedures and results. Copies of any questionnaires, data collection forms, letters of recruitment, information to participants, consent forms, etc., can be included in the appendices.

If a secondary analysis has been undertaken using an existing dataset, the sources of data or selection of material, steps taken to ensure the reliability of procedures and quality of data, and their fitness of purpose for your work should be addressed. If the methodology has been informed by theoretical perspectives of conceptual frameworks, this should also be discussed.

No results should be reported in the methods section. For example, although your proposed sample size should be included in the methods section, the number of participants actually recruited should be reported in the results section (see below).

Results

The content and structure of this section will be governed by the study objectives. For some studies, sections corresponding to results relating to each of the objectives may provide a suitable framework. If a questionnaire or semi-structured interview schedule was used, the results could be presented in question order. In a qualitative study, broad themes identified during the analysis of data may provide a logical way of organising the results section. The length of the results section will vary markedly between studies. For some quantitative studies, the findings can be effectively reported in a few tables with minimal supporting text. Conversely, qualitative work may require detailed discussion of respondents' perspectives on a wide range of issues, possibly drawing on established theoretical frameworks or policy statements.

The results section will often start with a report of the number of cases or participants included, the number or range of documents that you examined, the number and duration of observation periods or number of observations, the number and length of interviews, etc. This section may also include information on response rates, missing/completeness of data, unexpected events or any problems in the execution of the study.

A descriptive analysis of the dataset sets the scene for subsequent analyses. Knowing how many participants there were and their characteristics, such as age, sex, location of work, socioeconomic background, aspects of medicines use, and any other characteristics relevant to the study, is essential for the planning of the analysis and interpretation of results. Any available information on non-responders or missing data should be reported with, if possible, a comparison of responders and non-responders and assessment of possible bias. This will enable the reader to assess the probable representativeness of the sample. If relevant information is available, it may be possible to compare some of the characteristics of the sample with those of the wider population.

Quantitative studies

In reporting the findings in quantitative studies, tables, bar charts, histograms or pie charts can improve the presentation and aid the interpretation of the results. When these are used the accompanying text need not repeat the information in these tables and figures, but can be used to draw attention to important features or comment on and explain any apparent inconsistencies. The text can also be used to report and describe any associations between variables, and to summarise the findings in relation to each study objective.

Qualitative studies

In qualitative work the results and discussion sections are sometimes combined. This can be helpful to the researcher because data analysis is to some extent an interpretative process in which later stages of the analysis build on earlier ones. Points raised in discussion (theoretical perspectives or findings from the literature) may have informed and directed the analysis. In these cases, by combining the two sections it makes it easier to explain the rationale for the analysis and enables you to describe the results in the context of your theoretical framework. For example, if you wished to examine ways in which your findings support existing theories or hypotheses in the literature, you may have constructed your analysis to enable this investigation. It may be easier to incorporate a discussion of ways in which your data do or do not support this earlier work when presenting your results rather than having separate results and discussion sections, which can result in a lot of repetition.

A single results/discussion section will comprise the results of your study, discussion points identified in the literature (including results of other studies and/or theoretical perspectives) and your own thoughts on your findings (including bringing the results and discussion together). However, when combining the results and discussion sections, it must be written so that it is always clear to the reader when you are referring to your own findings and when you are drawing on other sources for comparison.

Presentation of the results in qualitative work is often supported by verbatim quotations. These are taken directly from the transcripts and so it is only possible for data that are audio recorded, transcribed word for word and for which the context is clear. As the aim of qualitative work is usually to present issues from the perspective of respondents, use of their words to illustrate the findings is seen as logical. However, quotations must not be a substitute for analysis and critical thought on the part of the researcher. The rationale for the selection of quotes must be apparent. A quotation may be included to represent, in context, a typical viewpoint, or to demonstrate a common problem experienced by respondents. A series of quotes may be used to illustrate a range of viewpoints or experiences, or perhaps to portray extreme cases. It is easy to find many interesting quotes, but it can be very challenging to embark on an in-depth analysis and interpretation of the data. Quotes should be selected to illustrate your findings and enhance the reader's insights into the issues. However, in terms of presentation of the results, their use should be seen as secondary and kept to a minimum. It is also conventional to attribute each quote to a respondent. It should be possible for the reader to see which quotations were attributable to the same respondent. Sometimes further information may be provided on relevant characteristics of the respondent; of course anonymity must be preserved.

Qualitative studies generally involve small numbers of respondents, who are purposively selected. Thus, reporting of numbers or proportions of respondents who hold particular views is usually not the intention. However, in some studies, it may be appropriate to inform the reader when a view was universally held or whether an issue was raised by only one individual. This information may provide insights into situational factors or contexts that might give rise to particular phenomena. Qualitative studies may aim to provide possible explanations for phenomena, e.g. a legitimate question may be: 'Could a particular experience or problem result from certain identifiable factors?' Thus, in qualitative studies the reporting of numbers of respondents holding particular views is sometimes helpful and justified.

As a general rule, in the results section of a qualitative study, all issues raised by respondents should be included. As samples are usually small, often with purposive selection of one or two individuals to represent a particular group, points raised by only one respondent are not necessarily less important. These issues may be pertinent to situational factors that were unique to that particular respondent. If a purposive sampling procedure were employed, there may be only one such individual in the sample, but similar situations may be replicated in the wider population.

Discussion

The content of the discussion will be determined by the study objectives and results. However, a few general thoughts will be relevant to most studies (*Box 16.1*).

The discussion can sometimes become a reiteration of the results, but it must not be. Avoiding repetition of the results (to facilitate their discussion) can be difficult. Perhaps the best way to avoid this is to have a clear alternative agenda for the discussion. The results should be taken as read, the discussion focusing on their implications. No new results should be presented in the discussion section. Depending on the objectives and topic area of the study, the following thoughts may assist you in developing a framework for the discussion:

- The specific objectives of the study: Comment on the extent to which these were met and the implications of specific findings for each objective.
- The literature, including previous studies and/or theoretical perspectives: Relate your findings to those of other researchers. Relevant work will have been identified during the literature review at the start of the study. Depending on the duration of your project, it may be necessary to update your review, to check for more recent work. Consider how your work builds on, extends, or contradicts existing literature on the subject. When comparing your findings with those of others, you should not report just any similarities and differences, but also comment on how any inconsistencies might be explained.
- Implications and recommendation for practice: Comment on the implications of your results for future pharmacy or broader healthcare services/practice in the relevant area of your study. This should answer the question of 'So what?'. What needs to change as a result of your findings?
- Recommendations for future research: Do your findings suggest any future projects that may be valuable to carry out? For example, if an

audit or service evaluation identifies weaknesses in the current services provided, does another project need to be carried out to find the reason for these and any barriers to improving standards or services?

- The policy context: If the objective or topic of study has direct (or indirect) relevance for some aspect of health/pharmacy/drug use policy. The findings of the study may enable recommendations to be made.
- The methodological strengths and limitations of the study: These should be acknowledged. Suggestions as to how they might be overcome, and what implications they may have for the results should be discussed. You should ask the question: 'Given the limitations of the study, are the conclusions really justified?'

You should make it clear to the reader what your work adds to the literature in the field and why it is important or valuable. You should not leave it to readers to work out these things for themselves. The discussion may end with a conclusion.

Box 16.1: Planning the discussion: some possible subheadings

- Summary of main findings and extent to which objectives were met
- Strengths and limitations of the study
- Comparison with previous research/literature on the subject
- Implications/recommendations for policy and practice
- Suggestions for future research

References

In identifying all your references and other sources you must be comprehensive. All sources must be included and correctly attributed. From the early stages of the project, when undertaking the literature review or preliminary fieldwork, you should maintain full records of all your references and sources (including personal communications) (see *Box 8.3* in **Chapter 8**). In constructing your reference list, you should be consistent in your style, providing full information in a similar format for each entry. It is best to use a standard procedure right from the start, such as the Harvard or Vancouver system (*Box 16.2*); most journals use one or the other of these. Following a standard procedure will help you to ensure that you are:

- comprehensive in identifying all sources
- consistent in your presentation of information on all sources
- complete in the information that you provide in relation to each.

Box 16.2: Harvard and Vancouver systems for referencing

- The Harvard system includes the names of the author(s) and date of publication in the text. The full citations are then listed alphabetically in the reference section. If there are more than two authors, generally only the first will appear in the text followed by *et al*. The names and initials of all authors will be cited in the reference section.
- The Vancouver system is a numbering system. In the text numbers are used sequentially at each point to be referenced. The reference section then lists in numerical order the full references in order of appearance in the text.

Appendices

The appendices should be numbered according to the order in which they are referred to in the project report. They may include copies of letters sent to potential participants, information leaflets/consent forms, questionnaires, interview schedules, data collection forms and any other study instruments or documentation that may be of interest to the reader. In some cases, additional, usually more detailed, analyses appear in the appendices, especially when these may be of interest only to specialist readers. When a maximum word count is prescribed for a project write-up or paper, this often excludes the title page, contents pages, abstract, references and appendices. Sometimes quotations are also excluded.

Conclusion

The project report needs to be written to a high standard, as once the work is complete it is on this that the project will be judged. The report should include a carefully constructed case regarding the rationale for the study, its methods, procedures and operation. The findings should be presented in a clear and logical way, with appropriate detail. The discussion and conclusions should demonstrate critical appraisal of the findings in the context of the methodology employed and the operation of the work, including the limitations. The contribution of the study to the existing literature and/or implications of professional practice or policy should be considered. The final report will also provide the basis for wider dissemination, which is an essential activity if the findings of research are to have any impact on professional practice, medicines use or service development.

Questions

1. Name the key sections that should be included in a research report.

2. Which one of the following is true with regards to the background section?
   A: The findings of previous papers should be presented without critique
   B: The writer should avoid drawing together the findings of individual studies
   C: Research aims and objectives should be included

3. Which one of the following should NOT be included in the methods section?
   A: The research design
   B: Justification of the methods chosen
   C: Sample size calculations
   D: Description of the sample recruited

4. Which one of following is true with regards to the presentation of research findings?
   A: Bar charts should always be included in the results section
   B: The text should draw out the key findings from the tables
   C: The sample size is not needed if a percentage is reported
   D: Quotations should form the majority of the results section for a qualitative study

5. Which one of the following should NOT be included in the discussion section?
   A: A summary of how the results meet the objectives
   B: Additional results, not presented in the results section, to aid in the interpretation of the findings
   C: Discussion of the results in light of the literature
   D: Reasons for differences between the study findings and the results presented in the literature
   E: Implications for practice
   F: Implications for future research

CHAPTER 17

Dissemination of the findings

LEARNING OBJECTIVES

Upon completion of this chapter you should be able to:

- identify key audiences to consider for dissemination of your findings in order to increase impact
- identify the media through which to consider disseminating your findings
- plan a presentation of your findings.

In addition to preparing a full project report, you may wish to make your findings available to other audiences. In many cases the research will have been undertaken with a particular application in mind and not just purely for educational purposes. People who have been involved in the supervision of the work or have collaborated in any way may like to see the outcomes. Funding bodies will be reluctant to provide resources for research unless they are convinced that the findings will have an application and value. A study may have relevance to just a local setting, or be of interest more widely. Dissemination is viewed as a crucial element in the research process. Researchers are expected to have considered how they will disseminate and/or publish their findings to ensure that they reach appropriate audiences so that they can inform future services.

It is common for research to be presented, in the first instance, to a local audience. This may be to fellow students, members of the department or institution in which the work was conducted, and/or to any individuals who assisted with the work or with a particular interest in the field.

Oral presentations

The level of detail to be included will depend on the length of time available. As a general rule you should aim to leave time for questions and discussion at the end, e.g. in a 15-minute slot, prepare a 10-minute presentation, allowing 5 minutes for discussion. In a 30-minute slot, a 20-minute presentation with 10 minutes for discussion would be appropriate. If you have 45-60 minutes in total, you could leave 15-20 minutes for discussion. You should rehearse your talk to familiarise yourself with the points that you wish to make (especially if these include explanations of relatively complex phenomena or procedures) and check that it falls within the time limits.

Oral presentations of research (whether to a local audience or at an international conference) are usually short. If you have spent several weeks, months, or even years, working on a research project, it will be a challenge to convey your important messages successfully in a limited time. You should also remember that in many cases your audience will be listening to a series of presentations, possibly on varying topics, in a relatively short period. The talk must be well organised and easy to follow, and kept as simple as possible while still maintaining the detail and depth required to convey the key messages, and assure the audience of their scientific validity.

Thus, the material to be included must be carefully selected. In a large project you may opt to focus on a single objective rather than attempt to cover all aspects of the work. If you decide to do this, your intention must be made clear to the audience and sufficient background and description of methods must be included. It may be at the results stage that you home in on specific aspects.

The presentation will usually be structured as introduction, methods, results and discussion/conclusions; all of which will necessarily be brief. The purpose of the introduction is to inform the reader of the reasons for undertaking the work. A few minutes at the start of the talk may be devoted to describing the problems to be addressed, highlighting any relevant policy issues and/or existing literature on the subject. The introduction often ends with a statement of the aims and objectives of the project. It should be clear how these will contribute to the subject area under study.

A description of the methods will then follow. This should include some justification of why particular procedures were selected, and the acknowledgement of any important shortcomings (as well as the strengths). The results of any study must be interpreted in the context of the methods used. Although you do have to be relatively brief, the audience must have some understanding of the methodological approach so that they can come to some independent assessment and interpretation of the results.

The results are usually the most important part of the presentation. These must be well organised and clearly presented. You may commence the results section with an overview of what you are going to present, e.g. you may present the findings relating to each objective in turn, or you may start with an overview of the main findings and then focus in more detail on selected issues.

It is important to be realistic about the range, detail and depth of information that can be included in the time available. You may have to be selective about what you can include. If graphs or figures are to be used, you must leave sufficient time for explanation of what they show and for the audience to make sense of the material for themselves.

The talk will usually finish with a discussion of points that you feel are important, conclusions relating to the study objectives and/or policy implications of the findings. You may have particular issues that you wish to highlight for discussion. Depending on your audience (e.g. if it includes people with particular expertise or experience), you may request their thoughts on specific aspects of the study procedures or findings.

Attention should also be paid to the presentation of material. Slides should be well laid out, and not congested with too much material. The size of print should be such that text, graphs and figures can easily be read from the back of the room. When presenting you should stand so that you do not obstruct the audience's view of the screen. The number of slides should be appropriate to the length of the talk and the complexity of the material, e.g. you could aim for an average of one slide for every 1-2 minutes of your talk (*Box 17.1*).

> ## Box 17.1: Suggestions for a 10- to 15-minute oral presentation
>
> - Title: one slide – affiliation, collaborators and date
> - Introduction/background: one to two slides – setting the scene and building the case for the study
> - Aim and objectives: one slide
> - Methods and procedures of study: one to three slides
> - Results: four to six slides – you may have to be selective in the results that you present, bearing in mind the interests of the audience, and maintaining clarity
> - Discussion/recommendations/implications: one to three slides

Poster presentations

These are a common alternative to oral presentations. At a poster session, the authors stay next to their poster for a set period and are ready to discuss their work or answer any questions. Many of the principles discussed above in relation to oral presentations will apply when preparing a poster. Posters are also often structured into introduction, methods, results and discussion sections (*Box 17.2*). Material under each of these headings must similarly be carefully selected. In terms of the level of detail, range of issues, etc., you should bear in mind that people may be viewing many posters in a single session, and therefore will spend no more than a few minutes at each. Material should be logically and attractively presented so that the essence of the study is easy for the viewer to extract; including too much complex detail may be off putting. You should aim to convey only a few simple messages in the body of the poster. You will be on hand to provide more information should this be requested. You could prepare leaflets with additional information for people to take away. These could also be used as summaries for dissemination to people unable to attend a poster session, but who have either had some involvement in the work or expressed interest in the project.

Remember posters need to tell a mini story of your project. If you are not presenting results relating to all your project objectives, then only include the objectives you are presenting in your poster.

Box 17.2: Suggestions for preparing a poster

- Include sections:
  - Title and your name and the collaborators, affiliations and contact details
  - Introduction/background: to set the scene and build the case for the study
  - A statement of aims/objectives or research question
  - Summary of methods employed
  - Presentation of results: often selected according to the interests of the audience
  - Brief discussion of their application or implications
- Think about the visual display
  - Overall organisation and layout
  - Inclusion of diagrams/figures/photos, as well as text
  - Use of different colours
  - Font sizes and styles
- Present clear messages that can be digested in just a few minutes
- You could also prepare a one- or two-sided A4 summary of your study with your contact details

Summaries for local dissemination

There is always a time lag (rarely less than a year) between completion of a study and the publication of the findings, so you may wish to prepare summaries of the report for dissemination to individuals who participated in the project, advised or assisted you with the work, and/or expressed an interest in the results. It is perhaps only courteous to acknowledge the interest and participation of others (especially those who gave their time and commitment) by keeping them informed of your progress and findings. The level of detail in the summary will depend on the intended audience.

Presenting at a conference

Local, national or international conferences provide important opportunities for the dissemination of research findings. Presentation at a conference often precedes publication. Conferences are usually organised with specific audiences in mind, e.g. they may be principally for researchers or practitioners or professionals from one discipline or across disciplines. The anticipated audience is often an important factor in your selection of a suitable conference. By presenting your work at a conference you can bring your work into the public domain more quickly than by publication in a peer-reviewed journal. Also, you will receive some immediate feedback from, and have an opportunity to discuss your work with, colleagues undertaking similar work or with interests in the same field. This may help you to identify other issues or perspectives surrounding your work. It may also help you to consider how you may approach publication, or plan to follow up your research. Discussion of findings at a conference does not generally preclude the subsequent submission of the research to a journal.

Conferences may be advertised one or even two years in advance, so you may want to be on the look out for an appropriate forum from the early stages. The first step in presenting your work at a conference is the submission of an abstract. Abstracts will usually have to be submitted to conference organisers about six months before the conference.

Writing a conference abstract

It is on the basis of the abstract that a decision will be made about whether or not to accept your work for presentation at the conference. Abstracts are brief (often one A4 page). Requirements for the structure vary, and it is important that you conform because the abstract, if accepted, may be inserted directly into an abstract book or the conference proceedings.

In writing the abstract it is helpful to follow an introduction, methods, results, discussion structure, even if this is not a requirement. The abstract is effectively a summary of the study prepared with a particular audience in mind. As a result of its brevity, the introduction will often be confined to two or three sentences, although the aims and objectives must be clear. The methods will also be brief but should communicate key information such as type of study (e.g. quantitative or qualitative), study setting, sampling procedure and sample size, and principal methods of data collection, processing and analysis. An overview of the results should be included; however, space will permit only limited detail and this is all that will usually be expected. The abstract should conclude with a comment on the important findings and their implications. The abstract as a whole needs to stand alone and present a mini overview of your findings; for example, the conclusion will follow on from the results presented.

The content of the abstract (and hence the material to be presented) will be influenced by the conference audience, e.g. the messages and focus of your talk will depend on whether you are addressing a group of researchers, health professionals, students, patients, policymakers or others.

The selection of abstracts by the conference organisers will frequently follow a peer-review process. The abstracts will be forwarded to members of a scientific committee who will comment on their suitability for presentation at the conference. The criteria used in this assessment are sometimes published in advance, but often include the scientific validity of the research and relevance to the conference themes and audience.

At many conferences research is presented in both oral and poster sessions. You may have the opportunity to express your preference. Some guidance on the choice of oral or poster presentation and their preparation is provided previously.

Papers for publication

Publication of their research in a paper is a goal to which researchers aspire. Publication in a relevant journal should be considered for research that provides new information or insights, contains important messages for practitioners, policymakers or other bodies, and is carried out to a high standard.

The first step is to decide which journal would be most appropriate. If the research was addressing issues relevant to pharmacy practice and the messages were for pharmacists, you could choose a pharmacy journal. If the focus was on other aspects of drug use or clinical practice you might consider an interprofessional or more clinical journal. It is sensible to send the work to a journal where research into similar topic areas has previously been published because this may be a place where people with an interest in that field expect to find, and therefore regularly look for, recent work. You may also decide whether the study is relevant to a local, national or international audience.

Your decision about where to submit for publication may also be governed by the type of paper that you wish to write. Some journals are dedicated to academic research with an emphasis on methodology, whereas others (although still seeing rigour in methodology as important) focus on work that has an explicit application, e.g. relevance to health policy or professional practice. You may decide that, rather than prepare an academic paper, you would prefer to write a more informal article or commentary based on the project and its findings.

A research paper will comprise an abstract, followed by introduction, methods, results and discussion sections. All journals publish 'instructions for authors' which state their more specific requirements. The project report may provide a framework for a paper. However, some restructuring will be required to ensure that the focus of the paper is relevant to the journal's readership and conforms to their house style. Sometimes additional literature work or data analysis will be required.

After submission, it is usual for the paper to undergo peer review. The editor will send copies of the paper to independent researchers, who will be asked to comment on issues such as the subject area of the paper and the originality of the work, the methodological rigour, importance of the findings, validity of the conclusions, suitability for the journal's readership, and whether or not they would recommend publication. The editor will then make a decision on whether or not to accept the paper. The reviewers' comments are sent to the authors. If the paper is accepted, it is common for this to be conditional upon some revision in accordance with the suggestions and recommendations of the reviewers. After acceptance for publication there will often be a delay of several months before the paper appears in print. Before publication a copy of the proofs is usually sent to the corresponding author for a final check. Publication of research is a protracted process. A year from submission to publication is not atypical.

Webinars

Webinars are being increasingly used to disseminate research findings and allow for research findings to be presented to wide national or international audience without the need for travel. These may sometimes be recorded in a studio. However, more commonly the presenter(s) will present from their own computer in their office using a microphone and headset. Like oral presentations, these will usually consist of a set time for the presenter to present, followed by questions. Although the audience is not physically present, webinars still offer opportunity for interaction. In most cases questions will be submitted through 'chat' boxes and moderated by the webinar host.

Social media

Social media is an increasingly important part of disseminating research findings. Websites of affiliated organisations and Twitter are examples of places where you can highlight your research and signpost abstracts, papers and research summaries.

Dissemination to more diverse audiences

In addition to presenting to researchers, the research findings will be relevant and useful to others including patients, carers, healthcare professionals not involved in research and policy makers. Dissemination to these groups, with targeted messages of relevance to them, may increase the impact of your findings.

Dissemination to patients and carers

Material developed for dissemination to patients and carers should be written in plain English, avoiding technical language. It is helpful to have patient involvement in the development of these materials and to check its readability using an online tool. In addition to lay summaries, innovative ways of communicating findings to these groups may include short videos and infographics. Findings may be disseminated through patient and public engagement events, charities and patient groups. The Patient Association has a newsletter where it highlights research of interest to patients. Patients may have further ideas on dissemination routes and should be consulted.

Dissemination to practising healthcare professionals

Many practising healthcare professionals will not be present at conferences and are an important group to target; aspects of your findings are likely to be very relevant to them. Summaries and messages for practising healthcare professionals should be short and identify the key relevant findings. Many healthcare professional groups have their own practice journals, which should be considered; for example, *The Pharmaceutical Journal* may be suitable for publishing findings relevant to practising pharmacists.

Dissemination to policymakers

Policymakers are an influential group, and it is important to consider key messages for them which would increase the impact of your project. For this group in particular it is important to place your findings in the context of current policy. The *Health Service Journal* is an example of one aimed at policymakers. Local councillors, NHS Improvement, the Department of Health and the World Health Organization are also potential target audiences for your work.

Conclusion

The aspiration of researchers to have their work published in well respected journals is not misplaced. Researchers hope that their work will inform future practice and contribute to improvements in service provision, patient care and health outcomes. That research findings reach relevant audiences is of huge importance to funders who have limited funds and want to ensure that they are used for maximum impact. As a result of the short time frame, it is usually unrealistic to expect that projects undertaken as part of an undergraduate or Masters degree will lead directly to publication. However, the work is often important in that it may contribute to a wider research programme, the outcomes of which will be published or inform practice at a local level. Research that is not disseminated in any way is unlikely to contribute to current debates or influence service development. Proactively creating and carrying a dissemination plan is a key component of ensuring your research has impact.

Questions

1. **Which one of the following statements is true?**
   A: Project findings are likely to be too difficult for lay people to understand
   B: Pharmacy practice projects are unlikely to be of interest to those outside the pharmacy profession
   C: All student projects have the potential to influence future practice or research

2. **Which one of the following statements is true?**
   A: The conclusion in an abstract should be based on the findings you present in the results section of the abstract, rather the results of your entire project
   B: When creating a poster, you should include all your objectives, not just those that you have space to present findings on
   C: When creating a poster, you should use a small font size in order to be able to fit more of your research findings in

3. **Identify four audiences that you may wish to consider disseminating your research findings to.**

4. **Identify four types of media that you may use to increase impact of your research findings.**

5. **Write a plan for disseminating your project findings.**

Answers

Chapter 1: Introduction

1. **A, B, C, D, E and F**
   All answer options are correct. All of these are pharmacy practice research projects.
2. **Answer:** There is no definitive answer, but you might have included projects relating to pharmacy education, evaluation of pharmacy services, safety and quality of medicines use, staff workflow in relation to medicine prescription, dispensing and administration of medicines, pharmacoepidemiology, adherence and shared decision making regarding medicines.

Chapter 2: Types of pharmacy practice projects

1. **B**
   This is the correct answer as it is aiming to produce internal recommendations for service evaluation and further development. Identifying barriers to self-administration in the inpatient setting is more likely to be aiming to generate generalisable findings and produce external recommendations and therefore be classified as research. Testing the extent to which a self-administration policy is being followed in a hospital trust is likely to be classified as an audit as it indicates a specific measurement of performance against pre-existing standards.
2. **B**
   This is the correct answer as it indicates a specific measurement of performance against pre-existing standards. Determining whether there is an association between gentamycin dosing and nephrotoxicity is likely to be classified as research and determining the effects on the gentamycin dosing regime followed at a hospital trust on its patients' outcomes is likely to be classified as service evaluation.
3. **Answer:** A service evaluation will aim to produce internal recommendations for service development or improvement, whereas a research project will aim to generate generalisable findings and produce external recommendations.
4. **Answer:** The steps in an audit cycle are standard setting, collecting information relating to standards, analysing data to assess the extent to which standards are met, deciding interventions to implement and implementing interventions.
5. **Answer:** Effectiveness is related to how well the service works in terms of achieving its outcomes. Feasibility is related to the ease of service implementation, its workability and its acceptability.

Chapter 3: Setting up the project, protocol development and ethics

1. **Answer:** A project protocol is a detailed plan of all stages of a project: its conception, aims and research question, the methods and procedures that will be employed, anticipated outcomes and information regarding the timeline, costs/resources and management. The protocol should provide sufficient detail to allow a researcher to carry out the project and will be referred to and followed throughout its duration.
2. **Answer:** Specify the types of wards
3. **Answer:** Identify the time period which you are investigating.
4. **A, B and C**
   Answer options A, B and C are correct.
5. **Answer:** Patients may be identifiable from their initials. It would be preferable to use a numerical ID that is used solely for the purposes of the study.

6. **Answer:** If it is a rare condition and there are only low numbers of people at the trust being treated for it, it may be possible for others to identify participants from any information given about them, even if their names or initials are not used. Care must be taken in terms of who has access to any information that may identify them.

7. **Answer:** This would be seen as deception and would be unlikely to be considered ethical. Instead, other measures could be taken to reduce the Hawthorne effect. It could be recognised as a limitation and the results interpreted in the context of it (see **Chapter 13**).

8. **Answer:** It is only ethical for healthcare professionals to look at records needed for patient care, audit, service evaluation or research. They cannot view them for any other purpose or pass information on to anyone outside the care team or project team. You would need to explain this to your friend.

9. **Answer:** Before beginning a project, you should have an agreed protocol of what to do if this situation arises and follow this. If you have not agreed this in advance you should discuss it with your supervisor. While you are not directly responsible for patient care, there are ethical issues, and you may need to inform the care team and make a note of this.

10. **Answer:** Leaflets should be available in alternative formats such as large print, braille and audio.

Chapter 4: Time management and working with others

1. **B**

   Any deviation from the protocol that is proposed should be discussed and addressed by the full team. Unilateral decisions on the approach and methods by individuals regarding separate components of the project may undermine its integrity as a whole.

2. **Answer:** Typical milestones in a pharmacy practice project are completion of full draft of literature review, final version of protocol, preparation of Gantt chart, start and/ or completion of data collection, completion of specified sections of project write-up and submission of final project report.

3. **Answer:** To plan your project effectively, write a full project protocol and produce a Gantt chart. Review these regularly throughout the project.

4. **Answer:** Some potential factors that could prevent timely completion of your project include delay in obtaining approvals and slow recruitment. These may be mitigated by allowing additional time for these stages of the project and/or identifying potential alternative sources of data.

5. **Answer:** The answer will vary between projects, but stakeholders may include your supervisors, other researcher and healthcare professionals, patients, carers and members of the public. They will each bring their own perspectives to the project. Overall ownership will need to be taken by the student.

Chapter 5: Patient and public involvement

1. **A, B, C, D, E, F, G and H**

   All answer options are correct. All of these are activities that patient and public representatives might contribute to.

2. **Answer:** Consultation refers to one-off events where patient and public representatives are asked to give their opinions. Collaboration refers to ongoing partnership throughout a project. Patient- and public-led projects are run by patient and public representatives who ask researchers for their input.

3. **Answer:** Researchers can help patient and public representatives feel part of the team by: asking about their needs, experiences and preferences at all

stages, involving them throughout the project rather than for set activities, treating them as members of the team rather than separate from it, and providing feedback on how you have incorporated their suggestions, or why you may not have been able to.

4. **Answer:** Answers may include three of the following:
   - Misunderstandings and breakdowns in communication. These may be mitigated by very clear and precise communication at all times and also by being careful not to make assumptions.
   - Patient and public representatives have reported sometimes feeling overwhelmed. This may be mitigated by using a buddy system, checking in regularly with patient and public representatives during a study, avoiding the use of jargon, and ensuring that researchers' expertise is not allowed to dominate.
   - Researchers feeling criticised by patient and public representatives. This may be mitigated by recognising that the bringing and merging of different perspectives can add much value to a study.
   - Patient and public representatives becoming unwell, or those they care for needing increased care. This may be mitigated by finding out their needs, offering flexibility, allowing them to dial-in to meetings and being understanding if they need to step back for a while. Having a small team of patient and public representatives will help ensure there is continuous involvement, even at times when some representatives need to step back.

5. **Answer:** Answers will differ between projects but may include some of the following: development of patient information leaflets, development of the data collection tool, recruitment of patients, data collection, data analysis, monitoring study progress, and dissemination of research findings.

Chapter 6: For supervisors

1. **Answer:** Pharmacy practice projects can provide opportunities for students to spend an extended period in a professional setting, and to experience audit, service evaluation and research integrated into everyday practice. Supervisors have the opportunity to have assistance with a study that will support a wider research programme and/or answer questions that are pertinent to their professional practice.

2. **A, C and D**
   Answer options A, C and D are correct.

3. **Answer:** Strategies for ensuring good collaboration between supervisors may include asking the student to copy both supervisors into email correspondence, asking the student to send both supervisors notes of all meetings, and having occasional joint telephone meetings.

4. **Answer:** Some of the factors that could be taken into account to help a student plan their project are duration of the project, other student commitments during the project, approvals that need to be gained and any limitations on times that data collection can take place.

5. **Answer:** Creating a Gantt chart can help students with time planning.

Chapter 7: A scientific approach to your research

1. **Answer:** Taking a scientific approach enables you to step back and consider your 'world-view', the underlying assumptions and perspectives that surround your project and how these have led to the formulation of your research question and impacted on your conduct of the research.

2. **Answer:** Methods refers to how a project is carried out. Methodology is about the choice and selection

of particular methods to answer a research question.

3. **Answer:** There is no definitive answer, but you might have included your background, your experiences to date, your personal beliefs and your pharmacist perspective.

4. **A**

   Different students who are carrying out observations interpreting items on a data collection instrument differently would cause a reduction in reliability. Participants completing a questionnaire interpreting a question differently to how the researchers intended them to would cause a reduction in validity, rather than reliability.

5. **Answer:** Generalisability is the extent to which the findings of a study can be applied to individuals beyond the sample.

Chapter 8: Reviewing the literature

1. **Answer:** A scoping review provides a general overall broad picture of a research area, rather than an in-depth focus on a more specific area.

2. **Answer:** A systematic review will aim to systematically identify and critically review all literature that meets a set of predefined inclusion criteria.

3. **Answer:** Answers may include PubMed, MEDLINE, EMBASE, IPA, PsychINFO, IBSS ERIC, BNI and CINAHL.

4. **Answer:** Answers should include developing search terms, choosing relevant databases and developing inclusion and exclusion criteria. These should be linked to the aims and objectives of the review.

5. **C**

   The correct answer is that critical appraisal tools can act as a guide when critically appraising a study. When using critical appraisal tools, it may be that not all items are relevant

to your study. In general, these tools are best used as a guide to the areas of critique that may be relevant for different types of study.

Chapter 9: Study design

1. **A, B and D**

   Answer options A, B and D are correct. Randomisation, a control group and outcome measures are all features of a randomised controlled trial. Qualitative data collection may occasionally be carried out alongside a randomised controlled trial but is not a general feature of one.

2. **Answer:** A cross-sectional study is carried out at one point in time. A longitudinal study follows participants over a period of time.

3. **Answer:** Answers may include five from: case study, case control, cross-sectional, longitudinal (or cohort), experimental (such as randomised controlled trial), quasi-experimental (such as before and after).

4. **Answer:** A pilot study would be carried out to check that the project is feasible and will provide the information required to answer the research question.

5. **Answer:** Triangulation is the combination of different approaches, methods, and/or data within a single research study.

Chapter 10: Sources of information, datasets, sampling and recruitment

1. **Answer:** Primary sources are data that are collected specifically for the research study that is being conducted. Secondary sources refer to data that have been collected for another purpose, which may have been for a previous research study, or data that are routinely collected for monitoring practice, or other events and activities.

2. **B and C**

   Answer options B and C are correct. These will both result in random

probability samples. The other methods will result in non-probability samples.
3. **Answer:** A sampling frame is a list of all members of the population.
4. **Answer:** When determining a sample, researchers should take into account: the study design, the type of analysis to be carried out, the outcome measures used, the degree of accuracy desired when the estimate based on the sample is applied to the wider population, the anticipated response rate, the expected drop off rate and pragmatic considerations around the resource available. Power calculations may be performed to determine sample size.
5. **Answer:** There is no definitive answer. However, data sources may include databases such as The General Practice Research Database, THIN database or electronic medication records. Recruitment methods may include face-to-face, mailing, email or social media. Advantages and disadvantages will relate to the resource required, the type of participants being recruited, likely response rate and information that the researcher has about how the data was gathered and non-responders.

Chapter 11: Data collection – survey research and questionnaires

1. **D**
   Checking your questionnaire covers the data that is relevant to the objectives is a test for content validity. Measuring against a gold standard to check the degree of association is a measure of criterion validity. Testing whether participants give similar responses to questions one week after they first complete the questionnaire is a test of reliability. Checking your questions are clear is a test of face validity.

2. **Answer:** The question should be rewritten in a less leading way and split into two questions; one covering ease of comprehension and the other covering content. For example:
   Did you find the training:
   - very easy to understand?
   - quite easy to understand?
   - quite difficult to understand?
   - very difficult to understand?
   Did you find the training:
   - very relevant?
   - quite relevant?
   - not very relevant?
   - not at all relevant?
3. **Answer:** This question should be written in a less judgemental way e.g. Where do you keep medicines?
4. **Answer:** Categories of ages should not overlap e.g.
   - under 20
   - 20-39
   - 40-59
   - 60-79
   - 80 and over
5. **Answer:** The question should be less leading e.g. When do you take your tablets? A range of options could be given.

Chapter 12: Data collection – interviews and focus groups

1. **B and E**
   Answer options B and E are correct. These are open questions; the other options are all closed questions.
2. **Answer:** An advantage of focus groups is that the interaction between individuals may stimulate a wider ranging discussion and generate a more comprehensive list of concerns and issues important to respondents. A disadvantage is that some participants may be more dominant than others. In addition, some information may be sensitive, and participants may not wish to disclose it in a group setting.
3. **Answer:** Nominal group technique is a structured approach to group

interviews that is used in consensus building. It involves several stages including silent idea generation, sharing of ideas, classification and grouping and ranking.

4. **Answer:** A researcher can increase validity of interviews by trying to avoid making assumptions about the respondent, allowing their own preconceived ideas to affect questioning, or asking leading questions in the interview.

5. **Answer:** An interviewer can develop skills in encouraging views from a range of participants. In some cases, a more structured technique can be used.

Chapter 13: Data collection – prospective methods

1. **Answer:** Prospective methods are those in which data are collected as events occur.

2. **A, B and E**
   Answer options A, B and E are correct. These are primarily prospective methods of data collection. Questionnaires and audits are primarily retrospective methods.

3. **C**
   Prospective methods can be quantitative and/or qualitative.

4. **Answer:** For observations, the biggest challenge may be the Hawthorne effect i.e. the effect of your presence on the individuals you are observing; changes to behaviour may be conscious or inadvertent. In any observation study it should be assumed that the researcher will have some impact. Other disadvantages may be the time-consuming nature of observations for researchers and the time-consuming nature of filling in diaries for participants; the latter may lead to incomplete data.

5. **Answer:** You could approach the Hawthorne effect in two ways: firstly, consider how you can minimise it, and secondly by taking steps to assess

its impact. Possible steps to reduce the impact of your presence may be to explain clearly the purposes of the study so people are not suspicious of your intentions, provide assurances of the confidentiality/ anonymity of data, and when collecting data make sure you are as unobtrusive as possible. In most cases the operation of the study and place of the researcher needs careful planning and discussion with staff.

Ideally some attempts should be made to assess the ways in which, and the extent to which, the findings of the study are influenced by the presence of the observer and the research process. Clearly, some activities are more likely to be affected than others. One way to assess impact of the observer is to ask participants at the end of the observation how they felt that the observer's presence changed their behaviour. In addition, information may be available from other sources (e.g. questionnaires or interviews) to provide some insights into the likely the validity of data. Observation itself is also sometimes used to provide some validation of data in other types of studies. For example, self-reporting in questionnaires is sometimes compared with similar information gathered by direct observation.

Data collection forms or diary entries should be quick and easy to complete. Giving clear instructions and limiting time periods of data collection and the level of detail may help increase reliability. Simple practical steps may make a big difference, such as providing a clipboard for display of the documents, ensuring an appropriate print size, attaching a pen, or in the case of a paper-based diary discussing the size of the paper or booklet and its layout. It is important to check that what you are asking participants to do is acceptable, not too time-consuming or difficult. Study procedures and data quality should be tested in pilot work. During the study it is a good idea to keep in contact with participants to check whether they are experiencing problems in adhering to the study protocol and to address any difficulties as early as possible.

Chapter 14: Existing datasets and secondary analyses

1. **Answer:** Answers may include previous literature, electronic prescribing records, established research databases, policy documents and media sources as sources of primary data.
2. **Answer:** Advantages of carrying out analyses of existing data may include it being less time consuming and that potential ethical issues of asking participants to take part have already been accounted for.
3. **Answer:** Challenges may relate to the quality of the data, particularly if it had not been collected with research purposes in mind. Specific quality issues may relate to comprehensiveness, generalisability, reliability and validity of the data. These can be mitigated by finding out as much information as possible about how the data was collected, critically reviewing the strengths and weaknesses of using the data in answering your research questions and interpreting your findings in light of any limitations.
4. **Answer:** Three examples of methods of synthesising findings from qualitative studies include meta-analysis, narrative syntheses and realist synthesis.
5. **C**
   Narrative synthesis can be used to synthesise heterogeneous studies.

Chapter 15: Data processing and analysis

1. **A**
   Number of years since diagnosis is an interval variable.

2. **Answer:** As you are carrying out a test of difference and both your variables are nominal, a chi-square test would be most appropriate. However, if the expected frequency is less than five cases in each cell, a Fisher's exact test can be performed instead.
3. **Answer:** As you are carrying out a test of difference and number of medication discrepancies is interval, an unpaired t-test could be employed. However, you would first need to check that the data was normally distributed. If it was not, a Mann–Whitney U test would need to be employed instead.
4. **Answer:** As you are carrying a test of association with ordinal data, a Spearman's rank test would be appropriate.
5. **Answer:** An inductive approach allows themes, ideas and explanations of phenomena to emerge from the data, whereas a deductive approach applies a predetermined framework to the analysis of data.
6. **Answer:** In the course of the analysis, the researcher may attempt to use the data to argue a viewpoint contradictory to the tentative conclusions or theories, i.e. the researcher will (acting as the devil's advocate) take a systematic approach to looking for examples in the data that do not fit with his or her hypothesis or conclusions.

   After data analysis, the researcher may collect additional data to verify a hypothesis or ask the original participants to comment on the extent to which they believe the findings accurately represent their experiences and perspectives. This could be in terms of their description, possible explanations and the complexity.

   Researchers may compare their findings with those of other studies (in the literature) or relevant theory to assess the extent to which they are consistent. Where findings do concur, what does the study add? Where findings do not concur, what further questions are raised?

7. **Answer:** Two or more researchers may be involved in the development of the coding frame, possibly independently devising their own structures, which are then compared.

As a check on the reliability of the coding process, it is common for this to be undertaken by two researchers independently for a sample of the transcripts. Any discrepancies in the coding must be examined and the coding frame revised to ensure its consistent application.

Chapter 16: Writing the project report/research paper

1. **Answer:** The main sections in a research report or paper are the abstract, introduction, methods, results, discussion, conclusion, acknowledgements and references.

2. **C**
   Research aims and objectives should be included in the background section of a research paper/report.

3. **D**
   A description of the sample recruited should be included in the results rather than the methods section.

4. **B**
   The text should draw out the key findings from the tables in the results section.

5. **B**
   Additional results, not presented in the results section, should not be presented in the discussion section.

Chapter 17: Dissemination of the findings

1. **C**
   All student projects have the potential to influence future practice or research.

2. **A**
   The conclusion in an abstract should be based on the findings you present in the results section of the abstract, rather the results of your entire project.

A poster should tell its own mini story; only objectives relevant to the data being presented should be included.

3. **Answer:** Answers may include academic researchers, patients, carers, healthcare professionals and policymakers.

4. **Answer:** Answers may include papers, posters, oral presentations, webinars, videos and infographics.

5. **Answer:** There is no comprehensive answer as this will depend on the project. However, answers may include the audiences to which you wish to disseminate your work, the key messages for each audience, and the best way of reaching them.

Index

abstract for conference, dissemination of findings, 212
abstract/summary, project reports, 196
acknowledgements, project reports, 197
aims
  and objectives, 21
  protocol, 22
analysis, data. *See* data processing and analysis
anthropologist, scientific approach, 61
appendices, project reports, 197
audit, 13–16
  design, 90
  scientific approach, 64

case-control studies, 94
case studies, 94
  observation, 154
  qualitative research, 185
  research design, 98
categorical variables, associations between, 179
closed questions
  interviews, 141
  questionnaires, 126
coding frames and coding
  qualitative research, 185
  quantitative research, 171
collaboration. *See* working with others
comprehensiveness of data, existing datasets, 71
conclusion
  project reports, 197
conference abstract, dissemination of findings, 212
conference presenting, dissemination of findings, 212
confidentiality, ethics, 25
constant comparison, 186
  qualitative research, 185
constructing, questions
  cluster samples, sampling, 106
content and organisation, project reports, 196
contents page, project reports, 204
content validity, 124
critical appraisal, literature review, 75
cross-sectional studies, research design, 91
cross-tabulation, data analysis, 179

data analysis, 169. *See* data processing and analysis
databases, literature review, 76
data collection
  diaries, 158
  focus groups, 192

forms, 154
Internet/email, 134
interviews, 133
non-participant observation, 154
observation, 154
participant observation, 155
prospective methods, 154
questionnaires, 171
telephone, 133
data entry
  quantitative research, 174
data maintained by organisations, existing datasets, 164
data management, qualitative research, 190
data processing and analysis, 169
  approaching the analysis, 174
  categorical variables, associations between, 179
  coding frames and coding, 171
  constant comparison, 186
  data entry, 173
  focus groups, 192
  inferential statistics, 183
  intervention studies, 184
  Likert scales, 184
  measurement scales, 184
  multivariate procedures, 182
  planning the analysis, 175
  procedures, 178
  qualitative research, 185
  quantitative research, 170
  regression, 183
  reliability, 190
  stages, 170
  statistical analysis, 174
  statistical procedures selection, 175
  validity, 190
  variables correlation, 182
  Wilcoxon's signed rank test, 180
datasets, existing. *See* existing datasets
data sources, 102
  existing datasets, 162
  literature as secondary data source, 165
  literature review, 74
  questions, 102
data synthesis, existing datasets, 165
descriptive studies, 90
  research design, 91
  statistical procedures selection, 175
design, research. *See* research design
diaries, data collection, 158
disciplinary approaches, scientific approach, 62
discussion, project reports, 202

dissemination of findings, 207
  abstract, conference, 212
  conference abstract, 212
  conference presenting, 212
  oral presentations, 208
  papers for publication, 213
  poster presentations, 210
  presenting at a conference, 211
  publication, papers for, 213
  summaries for local dissemination, 211
  webinars, 214
documentary sources, sampling, 110
drafts
  meeting, 53
  writing up, 197
duty to prospective participants, ethics, 24

economist, scientific approach, 62
email/internet questionnaires, 115
  sampling and recruitment, 114
epidemiological research, scientific approach, 66
epidemiologist/pharmacoepidemiologist, scientific
  approach, 62
established research databases, existing
  datasets, 163
ethics, 17
  approval, 18
  confidentiality, 25
  duty to prospective participants, 24
  Foster framework, 23
  goal-based questions, 24
  informed consent, 25
  research, 22
  rights of participants, 25
ethnography, scientific approach, 67
evaluation of services, research design, 94
evaluation studies, sampling, 110
evidence types, literature review, 80
existing datasets, 161
  comprehensiveness of data, 162
  data maintained by organisations, 164
  data synthesis, 165
  established research databases, 163
  literature as secondary data source, 165
  meta-analysis, 165
  reliability, 163
  validity, 163
experimental and intervention studies,
  sampling, 109
experimental studies, 92
  research design, 92
  sampling, 113
  scientific approach, 66
exploratory studies, research design, 92
external validity. See generalisability (external validity)

face-to-face interviews, 145
feasibility studies, research design, 94
focus groups, 137
  data collection, 147
  data processing and analysis, 192
  sampling, 112
forms, data collection, 154
Foster framework, ethics, 23
framework approaches, qualitative analysis, 186

Gantt charts, time management, 30
generalisability (external validity), 71
goal-based questions, ethics, 24
grounded theory, qualitative research, 186
group projects, working with others, 33

hypothesis testing, research design, 92

inferential statistics, data processing and
  analysis, 183
information leaflets, recruiting participant, 117
informed consent, ethics, 25
internet/email questionnaires, 134
intervention studies, 184
  data processing and analysis, 185
  research design, 93
  statistical analysis, 184
interviews, 137
  closed question, 141
  content, 144
  data collection, 138
  face-to-face, 145
  guides, 138
  layout, 141
  open questions, 140
  questionnaire, 146
  reliability, 146
  schedule, 138
  techniques, 141
  telephone, 145
  types, 138
  validity, 146
introduction, project reports, 198
invitation letters, recruiting participants, 115

learning objectives, 7
  Master's degree, 9
  supervisor, 48
Likert scales, 184
literature review, 73
  critical appraisal, 84
  databases, 76
  data sources, 85
  evidence types, 80
  finding relevant material, 76

organisation and review, 83
overview, 87
protocol, 19
record keeping, 82
search procedure, 76
search strategy, 76
sources, 85
stages, 75
supervisors, 49
writing up, 87
longitudinal studies, research design, 92

Mann-Whitney U test, data processing and
    analysis, 180
Master's degree, 7
    learning objectives, 7
    research skills, 9
measurement scales, 184
    data processing and analysis, 184
    Likert scales, 184
meetings, 53
    drafts, 54
    reports, 55
    supervisors/students, 53
meta-analysis, existing datasets, 165
methodological approaches, 66
    qualitative research, 66
    quantitative research, 66
methodology and method, scientific approach, 63
methods, project reports, 198
milestones, time management, 31
multiple response questions, questionnaires, 127
multivariate procedures, data processing and
    analysis, 182

nominal data (categorical data), 179
nominal group technique, 149
non-participant observation, 154
Non-probability sampling procedures, 107
non-responders, sampling and recruitment, 117

objectives, 7
    learning, 7
    protocol, 20
observation, 158
    case studies, 158
    data collection, 154
    diaries, 158
    non-participant observation, 154
    participant observation, 155
    qualitative research, 185
    reliability, 155
    time and motion studies, 158
    validity, 155
open questions, 140

interview, 140
    questionnaires, 125
    questions, constructing, 140
oral presentations, dissemination of findings, 208
others, working with. See working with others
ownership
    project, 32
    supervisors, 32

papers for publication, dissemination of findings, 213
parametric/non-parametric data, statistical
    procedures, 177
participant observation, 155
patient and public involvement, 37
    challenges, 43
    Levels of involvement, 38
    partnerships, 42
    roles, 40
payment, working with others, 32
pharmacy practice research, 6
    Master's degree, 6
    scope, 6
    skills, 7
    value, 6
phenomenology, scientific approach, 68
pilot studies, 97
planning. See also time management
    Gantt charts, 30
    milestones, 31
    supervisors, 32
    timelines, 35
populations, sampling, 103
poster presentations, dissemination of findings, 210
preliminary fieldwork, scope and purpose, 19
presenting at a conference, dissemination of
    findings, 211
primary research, recruiting participants, 114
probability samples, sampling, 105
problematic questions, questionnaires, 128
professional environment, working with others, 32
project reports
    abstract/summary, 197
    acknowledgements, 197
    appendices, 204
    conclusion, 204
    content and organisation, 196
    contents page, 204
    discussion, 202
    introduction, 198
    methods, 198
    qualitative studies, 200
    quantitative studies, 200
    references, 203
    results, 199
    summary/abstract, 197

title page, 197
when to write up, 196
projects
    audit, 13
    ownership, 49
    planning, 18
    service evaluation, 12
    time management, 30
prospective studies, research design, 92
    data collection method, 92
protocol
    aims, 21
    literature review, 19
    objectives, 21
    pilot studies, 22
    preliminary fieldwork, 19
    preparing, 18
psychologist, scientific approach, 62
publication of papers, dissemination of findings,
    213
public involvement, working with others, 34
purposive samples, sampling, 109

qualitative approaches, research design, 98
qualitative research
    approaching the analysis, 174
    audio recording, 144
    case studies, 157
    constant comparison, 186
    data management, 190
    data processing and analysis, 170
    focus groups, 185
    framework approaches, 186
    grounded theory, 186
    interview guides/schedules, 138
    interviewing techniques, 141
    interviews, 141
    methodological approaches, 66
    observation, 66
    reliability, 99
    scientific approach, 192
    software, data management, 190
    validity, 190
qualitative studies, project reports, 200
quantitative approaches, research design, 99
quantitative research
    coding frames and coding, 171
    data entry, 173
    data processing and analysis, 170
    methodological approaches, 66
    scientific approach, 60
quantitative studies, project reports, 200
quasi-experimental studies, 93
questionnaires
    advantages/disadvantages, 123

closed questions, 125
content, 124
coverage, 124
data collection, 122
developing, 123
internet/email, 134
interviews, 133
multiple response questions, 127
open questions, 126
organisation/layout, 132
problematic questions, 127
question structure, 125
reliability, 130
subjective and objective quantifiers, 127
survey research, 122
telephone, 133
validity, 130
views/attitudes, 128
questions, constructing, 140
    closed questions, 141
    interviews, 140
    open questions, 140

recruiting participants
    information leaflets, 117
    invitation letters, 115
    non-responders, 117
    primary research, 114
    response rates, 117
references, project reports, 203
reflexivity, scientific approach, 63
regression, data processing and analysis, 183
reliability
    data processing and analysis, 191
    existing datasets, 111
    interviews, 146
    observation, 155
    qualitative research, 190
    questionnaires, 123
    scientific approach, 68
reports, 196. See also project reports, meeting
reports/drafts, writing up, 196
research design
    audit, 90
    case studies, 90
    cross-sectional studies, 90
    descriptive studies, 90
    evaluation of services, 94
    experimental studies, 92
    exploratory studies, 92
    feasibility studies, 94
    hypothesis testing, 90
    intervention studies, 93
    longitudinal study, 92
    pilot studies, 97

prospective studies, 92
qualitative approaches, 98
quantitative approaches, 98
quasi-experimental studies, 90
terms, 90
theoretical frameworks, 96
triangulation, 98
research skills, Master's degree, 7
response bias, 109
response rates, recruiting participants, 117
generalisability (external validity), 71
sampling and recruitment, 101
results, project reports, 199
review, literature. *See* literature review
rights of participants, ethics, 25
roles/responsibilities, working with others, 34

sampling
cluster samples, 106
documentary sources, 110
evaluation studies, 110
experimental and intervention studies, 109
experimental design, 109
focus groups, 112
non-probability sampling procedures, 107
populations, 103
probability samples, 105
procedures, 105
purposive samples, 109
representative samples, 104
sample size, 113
sampling bias, 113
sampling error, 113
sampling frames, 107
saturation sampling, 114
simple random samples, 105
snowball samples, 104
strategies, 104
stratified samples, 106
scientific approach
anthropologist, 62
audit, 64
disciplinary approaches, 62
economist, 62
epidemiological research, 66
epidemiologist/pharmacoepidemiologist, 62
ethnography, 67
experimental studies, 66
methodological approaches, quantitative and qualitative research, 66
methodology and methods, 63
pharmacist, 62
pharmacologist, 62
phenomenology, 68

psychologist, 62
qualitative research, 64
quantitative research, 64
reflexivity, 63
reliability, 69
sociologist, 62
survey research, 66
validity, 69
viewpoints, 61
scope, pharmacy practice research, 6
search procedure, literature review, 76
search strategy, literature review, 76
secondary data, literature as sources, 85
data maintained by organisations, 164
data quality, 162
documents, 166
research databases, 163
simple random samples, sampling, 105
sociologist, scientific approach, 62
software, data management, qualitative research, 190
sources, data. *See* data sources
sources, literature review, 85
statistical analysis, 165
stratified samples, sampling, 106
students
learning objectives, 7
meetings, supervisors, 50
support, 48
subjective and objective quantifiers, questionnaires, 127
summaries for local dissemination, dissemination of findings, 211
summary/abstract, project reports, 197
supervisors
learning objectives, 48
literature review, 49
meetings, students, 53
ownership, 49
planning, 50
Survey research, 66
questionnaires, 122
scientific approach, 66

telephone interviews, 133
telephone questionnaires, 133
theoretical frameworks, research design, 96
time and motion studies, observation, 159
time management. *See also* planning
Gantt charts, 30
milestones, 31
projects, 33
timelines, 51
title page, project reports, 197
triangulation, research design, 98

validity. *See also* generalisability (external validity)
    construct, 70
    content, 124
    criterion, 131
    data processing and analysis, 192
    existing datasets, 162
    face, 131
    interviews, 146
    observation, 154
    qualitative research, 192
    quantitative research, 170
    questionnaires, 130
    scientific approach, 71
value, pharmacy practice research, 6
variables, 19, 194
variables, statistical procedures selection, 176
viewpoints, scientific approach, 61
views/attitudes, questionnaires, 124

when to write up, project reports, 196
Wilcoxon's signed rank test, data processing and
    analysis, 178
working with others
    group projects, 33
    payment, 32
    professional environment, 32
    public involvement, 34
    record keeping, 33
    roles/responsibilities, 34
writing up. *See also* project reports
    drafts/reports, 197
    literature review, 202
    supervisors, 55